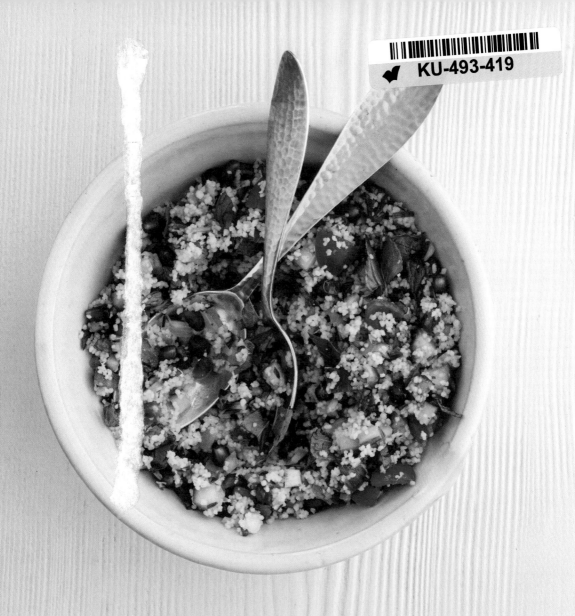

eat yourself

Pregnant

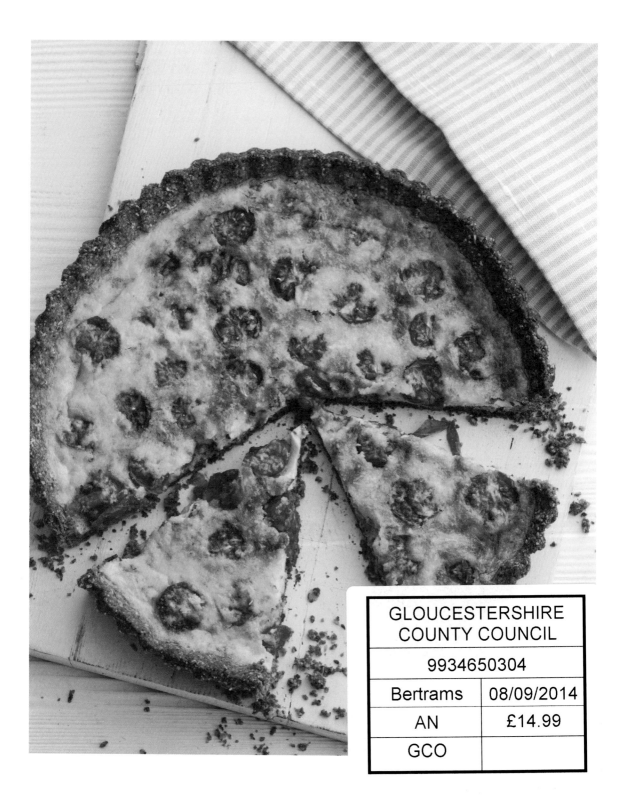

eat yourself
Pregnant

Essential Recipes for Boosting Your Fertility Naturally

Zita West

Recipes by Christine Bailey

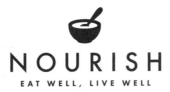

NOURISH

EAT WELL, LIVE WELL

Dedicated to my family – my husband Robert, daughter
Sofie and son Jack – for all of their help and support.

Eat Yourself Pregnant
Zita West

First published in the United Kingdom and Ireland in 2014
by Nourish, an imprint of Watkins Publishing Limited
PO Box 883, Oxford, OX1 9PL

A member of Osprey Group

enquiries@nourishbooks.com

Publisher: Grace Cheetham
Editors: Judy Barratt and Rebecca Woods
Designer: Luana Gobbo
Production: Uzma Taj
Commissioned photography: William Lingwood
Food Stylist: Bridget Sargeson
Prop Stylist: Wei Tang

A CIP record for this book is available from the
British Library

ISBN: 978-1-84899-207-8

10 9 8 7 6 5 4 3 2 1

Typeset in Caecilia and Calibri
Colour reproduction by PDQ, UK
Printed in China

Acknowledgments
My enormous thanks to Christine Bailey, who has done
such a wonderful job creating the recipes (and I am pleased
to say that I have learned to cook far better in the process!),
and to all my friends, family, colleagues and clients who
have tried them and given me feedback. Thanks also to
Matt Appleton, all at Nourish – Grace, Judy, Rebecca and
Luana – and to Bridget and William for making the food
look so wonderful. And thanks, finally, to baby Bailey for
the lovely cover photo.

Publisher's note
While every care has been taken in compiling the recipes
for this book, Watkins Publishing Limited, or any other
persons who have been involved in working on this
publication, cannot accept responsibility for any errors or
omissions, inadvertent or not, that may be found in the
recipes or text, nor for any problems that may arise as a
result of preparing one of these recipes. If you are pregnant
or breastfeeding or have any special dietary requirements
or medical conditions, it is advisable to consult a medical
professional before following any of the recipes contained
in this book.

Notes on the recipes
Unless otherwise stated:
• Use free-range eggs and poultry
• Use medium eggs, fruit and vegetables
• Use fresh ingredients, including herbs and chillies
• Use raw honey, where possible
• Do not mix metric and imperial measurements
• 1 tsp = 5ml 1 tbsp = 15ml 1 cup = 250ml

Watkins Publishing Limited is supporting the Woodland
Trust, the UK's leading woodland conservation charity, by
funding tree-planting initiatives and woodland maintenance.

nourishbooks.com

Contents

Key to symbols

D	Digestive boost
B	Blood-sugar balance
A	Acid–alkaline balance
E-F	Egg friendly (female hormone balancers)

S-F	Sperm friendly (male hormone balancers)
I	Immune modulation
S	Stress relief
L	Libido boost

Introduction

As a practising midwife and fertility expert, I have always been fascinated by the role nutrition takes in every couple's ability to have a healthy, happy baby.

My research and experience has shown me that good, wholesome food (and supplements as necessary) forms the bedrock of getting your body baby-ready and of making healthy eggs and sperm. Over the course of my many years in this field, I have come to the conclusion that micronutrients play a big role in getting pregnant – both naturally and through assisted conception – with deficiencies having significant effects on fertility for both men and women.

However, I also think that couples who want to make a baby need to have treats. Who could live without bread, chocolate, cheese and dairy? Not me! Whether you are just embarking upon trying for a baby, have been trying for a while without success, or have been diagnosed with a fertility problem, I want to reassure you that my philosophy is simple. Strict or faddy diets involve too many restrictions – they make what is the most normal and natural thing in the world seem strange and unfamiliar. My focus is on nourishing your body in a positive, sustainable way most of the time – not on challenging you to be 100 per cent perfect. I believe that small changes that are manageable within the context of your everyday life are all that you need. Quite simply, your pre-conception diet has to fit in with your 'normal' life or you won't be able to keep it up. Small steps can go a long way.

When I was first asked to do this book, I thought a lot about what happens in consultations at my clinic. I am very aware that many of the issues that come between a couple – just when they need most to be together – relate to lifestyle. I particularly see the contention that can build up around what food and drink lands on the supper table. I often find that one partner is trying to be too rigid, while the other wants to take a more relaxed approach. I think everyone can be happy – and that the resulting togetherness can only mean that you create more chances of making a baby.

Over the years, I have been so lucky to work with many wonderful fertility health practitioners, doctors, specialists in integrated medicine and nutritionists. All of them have had something important to teach me. However, the biggest impact on me has been the result of my work with Dr Stossier at the Mayr Clinic. There, the approach to fertility is integrated – modern medicine combined with the principles of Traditional Chinese

Medicine. Most importantly, this approach has taught me of the need for balance between all the body's systems – if one system is out of kilter, there is a ripple effect that touches every aspect of your well-being, including your fertility. Furthermore, I think the connection between mind and body has a huge role to play in a couple's ability to conceive, which is why I think it's important that your lifestyle choices are good and healthy, but also make you happy.

When I first meet a couple, I want to find out about the following things – their digestion and gut health, toxicity, acid–alkaline balance and immunity, and how much their states of mind are affecting their bodies. Only then can I begin to advise them on how to balance all these aspects of themselves to make the journey to parenthood a successful one.

This book is intended to inspire you and your partner to build on your excitement to create the best possible conditions for having a baby. The recipes have been carefully designed not only to taste amazing but to optimize your nutrition, too. Before you start cooking, read the first chapter for a thorough understanding of your aims, then leap into this journey together. I am sure you will find every recipe a pleasure to cook and eat.

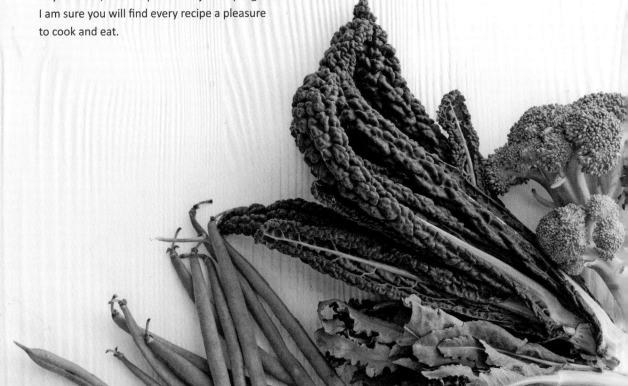

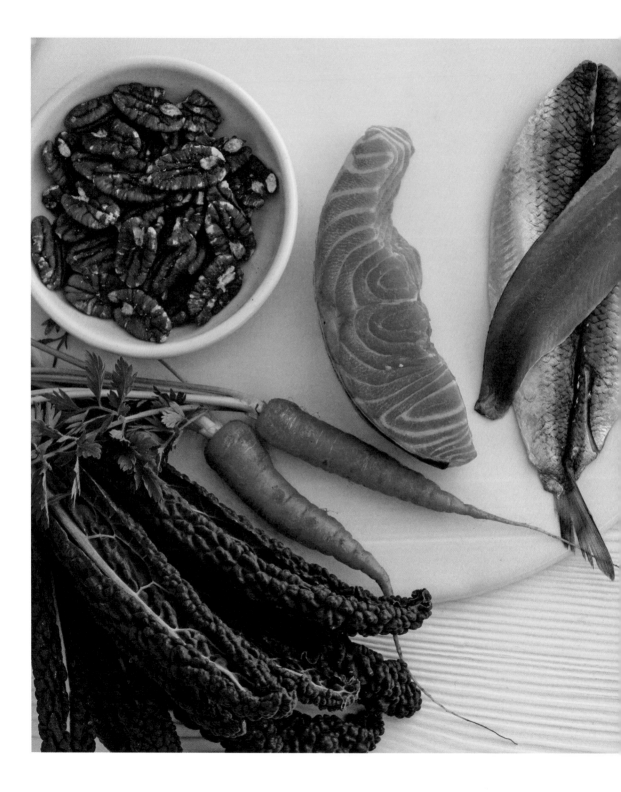

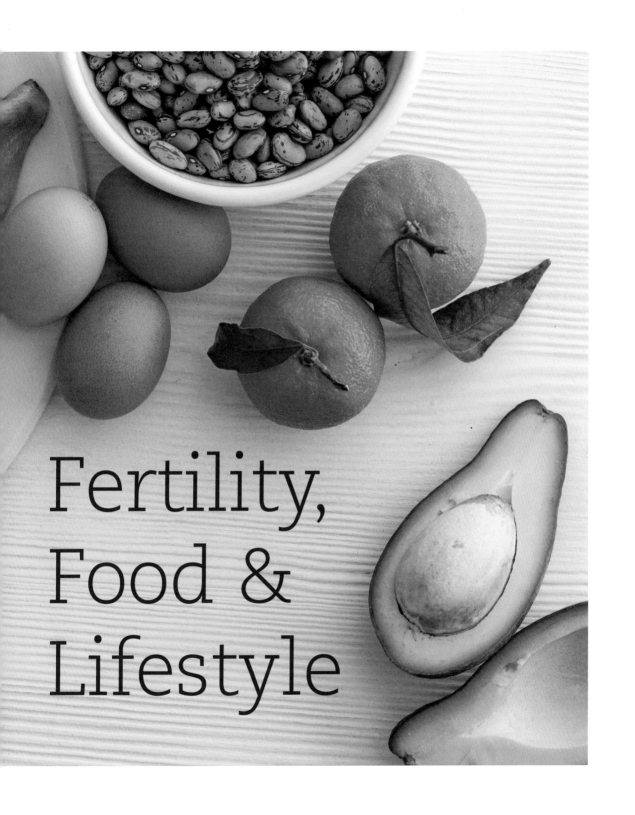

Fertility, Food & Lifestyle

The chemistry of babymaking

We all talk about 'romantic' chemistry – the magical, indefinable connection between two people that (when the time is right) may find its ultimate expression in a decision to have a baby. Then begins a whole new kind of chemistry – the chemistry of babymaking.

At the heart of this chemistry are your hormones – sophisticated chemicals that not only have regulated key stages of your physical development since the moment you were born, but continue to help your body to respond to its environment and to govern your fertility. Creating something as complex as a responsive human being requires an extraordinary degree of coordination, control and synchronization between these hormones. You need some other vital ingredients, too:

• healthy sperm
• a healthy egg
• healthy fertilization
• healthy implanation
• a healthy pregnancy

The chemistry of motherhood

During their reproductive years, women are ruled by a complex interplay of hormones designed to set up optimum conditions for pregnancy. Every month the hormones in a woman's body combine to create the menstrual cycle.

The first phase in the menstrual cycle is the follicular phase, in which follicle-stimulating hormone (FSH) primes follicles in the ovaries containing immature eggs to prepare for maturation. At the same time, the level of the hormone oestrogen rises, stimulating the maturation of one egg (sometimes more) and the production of secretions that will help sperm swim up the fallopian tubes (which run from the womb toward the ovaries) to reach the egg.

During the second, ovulation phase, oestrogen levels reach their upper limit, the egg finally matures and levels of FSH fall. At this point, the body produces higher amounts of luteinizing hormone (LH), which triggers the rupturing of the ovarian follicle so that it releases the egg. This is the point we call ovulation.

The third, or luteal phase, which in a healthy woman lasts at least 10 days after ovulation, is when the ruptured follicle produces the hormone progesterone to stop the production of FSH and LH and stimulate the womb lining to thicken in preparation for receiving a fertilized egg. If pregnancy does not occur, the level of progesterone falls and a woman enters the fourth, menstrual phase of the cycle – the period.

To produce a healthy egg, the right hormone has to be present in the right level at the right point in a woman's cycle. If timings are out of kilter or hormone quantities are too high or low, egg production can be affected. At its simplest, this might mean that pregnancy doesn't occur that month for no reason other than things were slightly out of kilter. At the extreme, hormonal imbalance can lead to irregular or no menstrual cycles and possibly other problems such as PCOS, thyroid issues, fibroids, endometriosis, and so on (see pages 22–3), which may have a detrimental effect on your chances of conceiving.

Other hormones

It's worth remembering that it's not just the menstrual hormones that combine to create the perfect chemistry for babymaking. A whole host of other hormones – some released from your brain, some from other organs – work together to create the best possible environment for pregnancy to occur. I've gone into detail about these on pages 16–19 – and many of them apply to fathers, too.

What makes a healthy egg?

The egg cell – or oocyte – is the largest cell the human body produces. It is 550 times bigger than a sperm cell. The egg cell consists of:

• **the plasma membrane** Situated around the cell, and composed of lipids (fat cells), the plasma membrane regulates the passage of nutrients and other material in and out of the cell.
• **the cytoplasm** This fills most of the cell and has sub-units called organelles, which carry out specific cellular functions. For example, organelles called mitochondria are the

Epigenetics – the chemistry of generations

While the genetic content of your baby's DNA is fixed at the moment the egg and sperm fuse, your baby's characteristics and even his or her susceptibility to disease depends upon the activation (or suppression) of particular genes during pregnancy. Epigenetics is the science that tries to establish what might influence how genes are turned on and off.

It seems that the environment in which the baby grows inside the mother – including what nutrients are available to it and what toxins are in the mother's living environment – will influence which genes become active and which do not. Most amazing of all, this influence not only affects the baby's own life, but also shapes the genetic make-up of generations to come. So, what you eat and how you live before and during pregnancy could have effects not just for your children, but for your grandchildren and great-grandchildren (and beyond), too!

powerhouse of the cell, providing it with energy; and lysosomes are tiny bags of digestive enzymes that break down waste materials and cellular debris and help keep the cell healthy.

• **the nucleus** Lying at the centre of the cell, the nucleus contains chromosomes that carry genetic material that will give the baby certain characteristics.

In order to be healthy, an egg needs the woman's body to provide:

• good hormonal fuel
• balanced blood-sugar levels
• good blood flow
• lots of antioxidants (and few free radicals)
• a good range of nutrients, including co-enzyme Q10, a fat-soluble antioxidant essential for energy production; B-vitamins, including folic acid, for the health of the egg cell's nucleus, its metabolism and its production of DNA (which carries our genetic material); and omega-3 essential fats and phospholipids for a healthy cell membrane. Furthermore, the egg is surrounded by follicular fluid, which also needs to be rich in certain nutrients, including vitamin D, betacarotene and inositol (see box, page 49).

Libido – the chemistry of two

It probably goes without saying that the desire to have sex in the first place – the libido – is essential in every couple's quest to make a baby. There are all sorts of circumstances and situations that can upset or enhance the delicate chemistry that affects libido for both men and women.

Time of day

Have you ever noticed how a man might be more passionate in the morning? This is because his testosterone levels (testosterone is the hormone of desire) are higher in the morning. If you're trying for a baby, I recommend harnessing all that early morning desire.

Closeness

Known as the 'hormone of love', oxytocin arouses the woman and primes her body for fertilization (and helps with bonding with the baby at birth). You can stimulate your body's production by encouraging closeness between you – cuddles, compliments and simple acts of kindness are all it takes to get oxytocin going.

Mood

Libido is greatly affected by mood. Emotions such as sadness, anger and frustration, and high levels of stress (including the stress of feeling under pressure to have sex around ovulation; and the increasing sense of pressure if conception doesn't happen quickly) can all lower levels of testosterone and oxytocin. Take a look at the box, opposite, for some ideas on how to eat to increase levels of feel-good hormones and keep the passion alive.

When and how often?

Perhaps surprisingly, many couples I see are simply not having enough sex every month to conceive. Mechanical sex or sex under pressure can have its own negative effects on your chances

Foods for mood and libido

By encouraging the body to produce certain neurotransmitters, or chemicals that act like neurotransmitters, some foods can influence mood and your desire for sex.

Dopamine This chemical helps us feel positive and motivated and is present in high levels during sexual excitement. The body manufactures it from the amino acid tyrosine in the presence of key nutrients including vitamins B3, B6 and C. Foods rich in tyrosine include chicken, lean red meat and turkey; cod, pike, shellfish and tuna; eggs and dairy products; avocado and bananas; and oats.

Serotonin This is the body's mood-booster. The body converts the amino acid tryptophan to make it. Tryptophan-rich foods include chicken, lamb and turkey; cod, halibut, salmon, sardines and tuna; asparagus, leafy green vegetables, potatoes, seeds and soya beans; and yogurt.

Phenylethylaminels. A mild stimulant, this is produced in your body as a by-product of the amino acid phenylalanine. It's the chemical that gives you that butterflies feeling when you first fall in love, making it great for reinvigorating the flush of desire. Chocolate is a good source of phenylethylamine.

of conceiving, but that doesn't change the fact that you needs lots of sex (especially at the right times) to have a baby. Lots, though, doesn't mean having sex every day (unless you want to). Aim to have sex three times a week. Don't worry if the mood doesn't take you more than that – sperm will last inside the woman's body for between three and five days. Women are most fertile in the five days leading up to ovulation, as well as on the day of ovulation itself, so do find your fertile window (see pages 24–5) and have sex at the right time of the month. The egg will live for a good 24 hours once inside the fallopian tube – giving it plenty of time to meet some sperm.

Couples often mistakenly feel they should be saving up the sperm inside the man's body and have sex only when the woman is ovulating. However, stale sperm is less potent than sperm that's been freshly made – so, sex throughout the month does make healthy conception more likely.

Finally, as an aside, lie flat for 15 to 20 minutes after sex; don't get up and go to the loo and don't put a pillow under your bottom. Also, don't worry if you feel that the sperm is falling out – it is a physiological occurrence called flowback and good sperm will make their way to where they need to go. In terms of your fertility, it doesn't matter if the woman doesn't have an orgasm, either.

The fundamental role of diet

Food – and all the things it's related to, from your digestion to your gut health – plays a crucial role in optimizing your fertility. This is where preparing to make a baby begins, at the basics – the way your whole body works.

Quite simply, the right nutrients give you the right building blocks for making a baby. What then should you and your partner include and eliminate in your diet in order to optimize your chances of conceiving? However, I don't want to be prescriptive; I think hard-and-fast rules are hard to stick to. Instead, I want to show you how nutrition and fertility are inextricably linked, so that you can make informed choices about your diet. Then, because your diet is one that you've carved out for yourself, you should be able to sustain it in the long term and so properly enhance your chances of conceiving. First, though, I want you to assess what your nutrition looks like now, so that you have a better idea of why and how you need to make changes. (Note that, when I say 'you', I mean both of you.)

How healthy is your digestion?
Fertility starts in the gut – the hormones you need to be fertile require key nutrients from the food you eat. Take a look at the following statements and answer true or false for each.
- I frequently burp or suffer with flatulence.
- I suffer from bloating and/or abdominal pain especially after eating.
- I suffer from irritable bowel syndrome.
- I regularly take antibiotics.
- I frequently suffer with constipation and diarrhoea.
- I have food allergies or intolerances.
- My stools are pale in colour or float.
- I frequently suffer with heartburn.

Answering true to four or more statements could mean that your digestion may be influencing your chances of conceiving. Look at ways to improve your nutrient absorption (that is, the health of your gut). You may also need a detox.

How toxic are you?
A considerable amount of evidence suggests that 'detoxing' – eating pure foods for a couple of days a week – helps to regulate hormones, lower cholesterol, balance blood sugar and improve digestion. To assess your present toxicity, answer true or false to the following statements.
- My urine is dark and strong smelling.
- I have bowel movements less than once a day.
- I suffer with headaches, fatigue, muscle aches and/or concentration problems regularly.
- Even one cup of caffeine makes me feel jittery.

- I drink more than 14 units of alcohol each week and sometimes I binge drink.
- My diet includes large fish such as swordfish, tuna or shark more than once a week.
- I regularly take medications, including pain killers.
- I drink bottled water from plastic containers, or unfiltered tap water.
- I eat lots of processed foods and foods containing lots of additives.
- I use chemicals such as those in some perfumes and cleaning agents.

If you answered true to five or more statements, you may benefit from a fertility cleanse. Take a look at pages 42–4 where I have set out a simple detox programme to prepare you both for pregnancy.

How stable is your blood sugar?

Your body breaks down carbohydrates (found in bread, pasta, potatoes, fruit juices, and so on) into sugars. These sugars are absorbed into your blood stream, triggering your pancreas to release the hormone insulin. High levels of insulin in the blood lead to fluctuations in your blood sugar, causing energy highs and lows, and in women increasing the production of testosterone – the so-called 'male' fertility hormone (see page 19). The resulting hormonal imbalance in women can affect ovulation.

To assess your blood-sugar balance, answer true or false to the following statements.

- I get jittery or irritable and I suffer from headaches if I skip a meal.
- I crave sweet things at around 4pm.
- I feel sleepy in the afternoon.
- I regularly wake in the night.

If you answered true to three or more of these statements follow the advice on pages 39–40. Integrate the recipes showing the blood-sugar balance symbol (see page 5) into your diet.

What's your acid–alkaline balance?

Although your body produces acids as a by-product of your metabolism, eating certain foods can increase your overall acidity. Too much acidic food in your diet places a strain on your liver and kidneys (your organs of elimination), leading to an increase in toxicity. The result is to deplete your body of nutrients vital for reproduction (among other things). In addition, sperm will survive longer in a slightly alkaline environment.

Have a look at the following list of statements. Answer true or false for each.

- I eat a lot of red meat and/or follow a high-protein diet.
- I eat sugary foods four or five times a week.
- I drink alcohol, fizzy sodas or caffeinated drinks four or five times a week.
- I eat fewer than two portions of fresh vegetables daily.

If you answered true to two or more of these statements, you may need to increase alkalizing foods, such as green leafy vegetables, in your diet. Read the advice on pages 40–1 and look out for the alkalizing icon (see page 5) in the recipes. Try to eat at least three of these dishes every week.

Your hormones, health and fertility

The reproductive hormones (those influencing the menstrual cycle in women and sperm production in men) represent just a small part of your complete hormonal system – called the endocrine system. The whole system needs to work in balance for optimum fertility.

Your endocrine system is made up of several glands and before we get into the detail of how nutrition can have a profound effect on your hormones, I think it helps to understand what each of these endocrine glands is, what hormones each produces and how each influences the reproductive system – as well as your body as a whole.

The hypothalamus and pituitary glands

Lying deep within the brain, the hypothalamus gland controls ovulation. It also influences the body's response to both internal and external stimuli, such as emotional and physical stress, and it triggers the release of the hormones FSH and LH (see page 10) from the pituitary gland, which is positioned below it. High stress levels inhibit the production of FSH and LH, which can interfere with ovulation.

The pituitary gland is also one of the sites in the body (there are several others) that produce the hormone prolactin. This hormone is best known for its control of milk production after birth, but prolactin also acts as a trigger, affecting the production of other hormones, such as progesterone, and can affect ovulation.

Together the hypothalamus and pituitary glands trigger the release of adrenocorticotropic hormone (ACTH). This messenger hormone tells other glands in the body to produce stress hormones such as cortisol and adrenaline, preparing the body for fight or flight.

The thyroid gland

A butterfly-shaped organ located just below the Adam's apple in the neck, the thyroid gland produces the hormones thyroxine (T4) and small amounts of triiodothyronine (T3). Hypothyroidism – a condition in which the gland does not produce enough thyroid hormones – is associated with menstrual irregularities and infertility.

People often underestimate the importance of thyroid function for fertility. The thyroid affects every cell in your body because it produces the hormones that regulate your metabolism. It adjusts calcium levels, fat metabolism, the way that oxygen is taken up in your cells and your weight – among many other functions and physical consequences. The thyroid's subtle effects throughout the body mean that an underactive or overactive thryoid can cause hormonal imbalances that may prevent

Stress and your hypothalamus

Your hypothalamus is your body's master gland that turns hormone responses on and off throughout your system. It is, therefore, the gland in control of your reproduction hormones – but it is extremely sensitive to stress. Poor diet and lifestyle and a life lived in a constant state of high alert tells the hypothalamus that ovulation needs putting to one side until a state of calm resumes. Quite simply, if your body perceives that you are in danger – which is what the stress response is for – it also thinks this would be a bad time to make a baby. To this end, pulses of follicle stimulating hormone (FSH) and luteinizing hormone (LH) cease, which means that oestrogen levels don't increase sufficiently to trigger ovulation.

It is my firm belief that stress management combined with following certain dietary principles, can make a significant difference to women who experience problems with ovulation specifically and with fertility in general. See pages 54–5 for advice on how to manage your stress levels.

pregnancy. If you have suffered two or more miscarriages, if your cycle is irregular or if you have a family history of autoimmune thyroid problems, ask your doctor to give you a blood test that will check your thyroid function.

The adrenal glands

Situated on top of the kidneys, your adrenal glands produce more than 50 different hormones, including the stress hormones cortisol, adrenaline, noradrenaline and dehydroepiandrosterone (DHEA), and the sex hormones progesterone, oestrogen and testosterone. When you experience a stressful event, your adrenals release adrenaline and noradrenaline to rapidly increase heart rate, blood pressure and blood-sugar levels to enable the fight or flight response. Ongoing, low-level daily stress, on the other hand, produces cortisol, a catabolic hormone that regulates blood sugar and the breakdown of carbohydrates, lipids and protein, and supports your immune system. Imbalanced cortisol levels can have detrimental effects on body composition, can lead to immune suppression and autoimmune conditions, and can disrupt the production of neurotransmitters and sex hormones.

The pancreas

Known as a glandular organ, the pancreas produces insulin in response to rising levels of blood glucose. Fluctuating blood-sugar levels (which can occur if you eat foods with a high

Could you be suffering from adrenal fatigue?

During times of stress the adrenal glands (see page 17) increase their output of the stress hormones cortisol and adrenaline. These narrow the blood vessels, restricting blood flow to the reproductive organs and so inhibiting fertility. However, the adrenals can't go on producing hormones at high levels – in the end even the glands get tired out, causing adrenal fatigue. This has its own problems for fertility, because of its effects on overall hormonal balance, mood, health and willingness to have sex.

Symptoms of adrenal fatigue include:
- chronic low blood pressure
- anxiety, depression and mood swings
- poor immunity
- increased pre-menstrual symptoms
- excessive tiredness
- feeling overwhelmed
- relying on coffee and other stimulants
- craving salty or sugary foods
- decreased libido

Do all you can to redress adrenal imbalance in your life. Certain nutrients can support the work of the adrenals. These include B-vitamins (especially B5) and vitamin C, the mineral magnesium, and essential fats. Try to 'create' time in your life: when you're eating, take time to eat; when you're thinking, take time to think; when you're working, take time to work. Spend time away from your desk doing the things you love – with the people you love – and even practise relaxation techniques (see pages 54–5). Above all, don't feel the need to fill the silences – let them be welcome pauses in your day.

glycaemic load, such as refined 'white' carbohydrates, potatoes and many breakfast cereals) can lead to increased insulin production. Over time, your cells can become less responsive to insulin's attempts at stabilizing your blood sugar, which triggers the pancreas to produce yet more insulin. Because insulin works synergistically with LH to increase the output of testosterone in your body, high insulin levels can lead to an imbalance in your reproductive hormones, in turn affecting fertility. The effect is worsened because high insulin levels also reduce the amount of serum sex hormone binding globulin (SHBG) in your system. SHBG clings to testosterone to carry it around your body to where it's needed. Women need some testosterone for hormonal balance, but if SHBG levels are too low, the amount of free testosterone (that is, testosterone that is not bound to SHBG) in the body increases, which can have a detrimental effect on a woman's fertility.

The ovaries and the testes

Finally, the endocrine system also includes the ovaries (in women) and the testes (in men), which are largely responsible for the production of your fertility hormones – oestrogen, progesterone and androgens (including testosterone).

Oestrogen

Oestrogen is produced in the ovaries in cells that surround the eggs. Rising levels signal the pituitary gland to produce FSH and LH when required. They also stimulate cervical secretions to assist the passage of sperm and the thickening of the womb lining (endometrium) ready for the implantation of an embryo if pregnancy occurs.

Progesterone

Once an ovarian follicle has released an egg, that follicle begins to produce progesterone to help the body prepare for pregnancy, including thickening the endometrium, blocking the production of FSH and LH, closing the cervix to prevent the passage of further sperm, and causing a slight rise in body temperature.

Androgens

Androgens, including testosterone, are produced by the ovaries and the adrenal glands in women and by the testes in men. They are important for healthy bone and muscle mass, alleviating depression, cardiovascular health and promoting sexual desire. Adequate levels of testosterone are important for sexual function in men.

The Hypothalamic Pituitary Ovarian Axis (HPOA)

The complex interactions between the parts of the endocrine system that regulate the reproductive cycle are referred to as the HPOA. The interdependence of HPOA hormones and the other hormones of the endocrine system has a cascade effect – as levels of one hormone change, other hormones have to adjust. In order for ovulation to occur, the delicate interplay of all the fertility hormones must work. Fertility problems, including perhaps no menstruation or ovulation at all, are often the result of an imbalance in the HPOA. Environmental or medical conditions, such as bodyweight, stress, drugs or PCOS, can all lead to dysfunction in the HPOA. Below are some of the most common fertility conditions I see in the women who come to my clinic – all are the result of an HPOA imbalance. The good news is that many of the causes of imbalance are correctable with the right diet and lifestyle choices.

Ovulation problems

The absence of ovulation – anovulation – is the commonest cause of infertility. It may occur, for example, if the pituitary gland fails to produce FSH or LH at the appropriate levels. The effects of stress on the adrenal glands, and hypothyroidism or hyperthyroidism, can also prevent ovulation.

Low levels of oestrogen are another cause of anovulation. Reduced oestrogen output may result from over-exercising or being overweight or underweight (see page 52) or, of course, ageing.

Using your diet for oestrogen balance

Oestrogen imbalance, which affects the fertility of both men and women, is increasingly problematic in the modern world. Foreign oestrogens are found in our water and in our soil (as a result of pesticides), and in materials such as plastic food packaging. One way or another, many of these leach into our food. (They're found in some cosmetics, too.)

Reducing your exposure to foreign oestrogens is one way to help reduce their impact, but it's also important to support your liver to help it detoxify them effectively.

Increase friendly gut bacteria

Your gut depends upon good bacteria, known as probiotics, to draw nutrients from your food and expel anything your body doesn't need. Live or bio yogurts, kefir (a milk substitute made using fermented grains) and fermented foods such as sauerkraut and miso are all rich in friendly bacteria. Take a probiotic supplement if you have to take antibiotics or are on the contraceptive pill, both of which deplete good bacteria in the gut.

Eat more dietary fibre

A high-fibre diet helps the liver because it encourages regular elimination via the bowel – preventing oestrogens from being reabsorbed into the blood stream.

Reduce saturated fat

A diet high in saturated fat – found in foods such as red meat and dairy products – limits the amount of oestrogen your body excretes.

Increase phyto-oestrogens

Natural compounds found in some plants, phyto-oestrogens exert oestrogen-like activity in the body. They bind to the body's oestrogen receptors, blocking them from receiving foreign oestrogens, so helping to restore balance to the system. (When ostrogen levels are too low their mild oestrogen effect raises oestrogen activity.) Sources of phyto-oestrogens include alfalfa, the cabbage family (including all types of cabbage, and broccoli, Brussels sprouts, and radicchio), chickpeas, cherries, dried apricots, fennel, garlic, hops, linseeds (flaxseeds), nuts, oats, olive oil, onion, parsley, prunes, pulses and beans, and seeds and their oils.

Increase vitamin B6

Low levels of vitamin B6 may make you susceptible to the stimulating effects of oestrogen. B6 also aids progesterone production. Food sources include avocados, bananas, cabbage (and the cabbage family), eggs, lentils, milk, molasses, soya beans, sunflower seeds, walnuts and wheatgerm.

How do I know if I have ovulated?

Many women worry about whether or not they are ovulating and use ovulation testing kits to try to gain some clarity. Although these kits will indicate whether or not you've had a surge of LH, so pinpointing the two days with the highest probability of conception, they predict only a short window and they can't tell you for certain whether or not your hormone surge actually resulted in ovulation. I also find that many women worry unnecessarily if the kits show no surge at all. Not detecting a surge may not mean you have not ovulated that month – just that your calculations for your cycle may be out. Read pages 24–5 for advice on how to monitor your cycle accurately and calculate your fertile time naturally. If your cycle calculations are accurate and the kits still do not detect a surge, you may have some other condition – such as PCOS (see page 22) – and you should consult your doctor.

Finally, having a period does not confirm that you have ovulated either. The only way to be absolutely certain that you've ovulated is to have a blood test for progesterone (see page 19) during the luteal phase of your cycle, or to fall pregnant.

Finally, if you've been taking the contraceptive pill, although you may be more fertile in the immediate months after you stop taking it, you may also experience cycle disturbances for up to nine months, while regular ovulation kicks in again. Although having a period is not necessarily a sign that you've ovulated, if you do come off the Pill and your periods do not return within six weeks, see your doctor.

Implantation problems

Progesterone dominates the second half of your menstrual cycle. It makes the womb lining thick and spongy, ready to receive the fertilized egg and provide the support necessary to maintain a pregnancy. If for some reason the ruptured ovarian follicle (known as the corpus luteum) fails to produce progesterone in the right amounts, the womb lining won't thicken and implantation can't occur.

If implantation does occur, but progesterone levels don't remain high, the womb lining comes away resulting in a very early stage miscarriage – one that occurs usually well before the woman realizes she was pregnant in the first place. Progesterone deficiency is very common, and in itself it may not be something to worry about. However, it may also signal that you are likely to be deficient in other hormones important for your fertility, too.

Eating for ovulation

I always think how magnificent a human egg looks when I see images of it – large, regal and ready for the sperm. The egg needs both nutrients and energy to prepare it for fertilization and to make its journey to the uterus. Surrounding your ovarian follicles is a follicular fluid that contains hormones and nutrients that nourish the egg before it leaves the ovary. However, this fluid can also contain free radicals that can harm the egg. So, above all, healthy eggs need lots of antioxidant foods (see box, page 33), which neutralize the effects of free radicals. Then, the natural compound myo-inositol (see box, page 49) may help improve the follicular environment and egg quality and to help balance blood sugar. Foods rich in inositol include beans, brown rice, lentils, cantaloupe melon, citrus fruit, nuts and seeds so make sure you include plenty of these in your diet, too.

Polycystic ovaries (PCO) and Polycystic ovarian syndrome (PCOS)

These are two distinct conditions. If you suffer from PCO, follicles in your ovaries have failed to develop properly and have instead become cysts containing immature eggs. Many women with PCO have no problems with fertility at all, although the condition is associated with raised levels of LH, which may damage the egg. PCOS, however, is an endocrine disorder and the resulting hormonal imbalance may affect a woman's chances of conceiving.

There are varying degrees of severity in PCOS, but the underlying cause is thought to be the ovaries' inability to produce hormones in the right proportions. Being overweight, having too many free androgens (see page 19), fluctuating blood-sugar levels and genetics are other causes.

A woman with PCOS is likely to have cycles that are longer than 35 days (oligomenorrhoea) or a total lack of periods (amenorrhoea) for four to six months. Excessive facial or body hair (hirsutism), male-pattern baldness, decreased sex drive, skin tags, acne, depression and a tendency to put on weight are all symptoms of PCOS. Blood tests will show high levels of LH and testosterone. Although the condition is not treatable, it is manageable and with careful attention to diet and lifestyle, many women with PCOS go on to have babies.

Endometriosis

This condition causes the endometrial tissue from the womb (the womb lining) to migrate to other parts of the body – generally the pelvic area, ovaries, fallopian tubes, colon and bladder. During the monthly menstrual cycle, the migrated patches of womb lining bleed at the same time as the womb lining itself, causing scarring and adhesions. The overall result is that a hormonal imbalance occurs, which in turn can affect a woman's fertility.

Many women show no symptoms of endometriosis at all, but for those who do, symptoms may include severe pain during intercourse, abnormal pelvic pain, heavy or painful periods or mood swings. The condition has various grades of severity (from mild to severe), so see your doctor for assessment.

Fibroids

Benign tumours that grow in the cavity of the uterus, fibroids do not always cause an imbalance in the HPOA. Whether or not they do depends upon where they are situated and how big they grow. Heavy periods, menstrual cramps, pelvic pain, or a sensation of fullness or pressure in the pelvic area are all common symptoms. Because fibroids are oestrogen-sensitive, managing your hormones can often deal with them effectively. They are particularly common in black women.

Hormonal balance and imbalance in men

In men, the testes are responsible for producing androgens – male fertility hormones that include testosterone, which every man needs in order to produce sperm.

One of the most important factors that affects testosterone balance is the amount of an enzyme called aromatase that circulates in the male body. This enzyme, which may be found in many of the body's tissues, including the gonads, converts testosterone to oestrogen. As far as male fertility is concerned, increased levels of oestrogen and reduced levels of testosterone can affect erectile function and libido.

Testosterone is not produced in isolation of all other elements in the endocrine system – LH (from the pituitary gland) triggers its production. Sperm production also relies upon another pituitary hormone – FSH (even though men don't have actual follicles). Sexual arousal, including but not limited to achieving an erection, relies upon the stress hormones (from the adrenal glands) and the hormones of the hypothalamus. Any imbalance in these and all the other hormones of the man's body can have an effect on his fertility.

Addressing hormonal imbalance

So, if all these conditions can cause hormonal imbalance that may affect your chances of getting pregnant, what can be done to redress the balance? There is no ideal substitute for a hormone that may be lacking, but there are certain nutrients – known as hormone precursors – that trigger hormone production. An optimal intake of key vitamins and minerals can therefore go a significant way to boost hormone production as necessary (so look out for the male and female hormone-balance icons on the recipes). And because boosting the production of one hormone can have the opposite effect on another, when certain hormones are operating at levels that are too high for optimum fertility, it is possible to use nutritional intake to lower levels, too.

How to chart and assess your fertility

Although there are certain parameters for a normal menstrual cycle, there are also many variables. Whether you're just beginning this journey or you've been trying for a baby for a while, understanding your cycle is a crucial first step towards eased conception.

So many of the couples I see are a little hazy on the nature of the woman's cycle. Here, I want to show you how to chart your cycle and your fertile signs so that you can optimize your chances for conception and, if relevant, have a better understanding of whether or not there may be a fertility problem. Every woman's monthly fertile window is different, and may even vary from month to month in the same woman. In general, though, there are five or six fertile days each month. These are the four or five days before ovulation and the day of ovulation itself.

Calculating your cycle

Before you do anything else, you need to work out the length of your cycle – from the first day of your period to the last day before the start of your next period. In most cases, it's more important that your cycles follow a pattern than that they are a certain length. To establish your pattern, chart your periods for six months, or longer if you have just come off the Pill (it can take up to nine months for regular cycles to return, although you may very well be fertile during this time). Any variation in cycle length within seven days is considered normal.

Most women ovulate 14 days before the end of their cycle, although ovulation could occur between 10 and 16 days (you need at least 10 days, as that allows time for implantation should your egg have been fertilized) before your period. If your cycle is 25 days long, and assuming you ovulate around 14 days before your next cycle begins, ovulation occurs typically around day 11; a cycle of 35 days means ovulation is around day 21; and for a much longer cycle of 42 days, ovulation occurs around day 28. Allowing for cycle variations (that is, differences from month to month), you can calculate that your six fertile days occur between the shortest cycle minus 20 days and the longest minus 10.

For example, if over the last six months your cycles have been 28, 26, 31, 25, 32 and 31 days, the shortest cycle is 25 days and the longest cycle is 32 days. So taking 20 from 25 gives you the earliest possible fertile day as Day 5 of your cycle (Day 1 is the first day of your period). Then subtracting 10 from 32 gives you Day 22 as your latest possible fertile day. So, you would be potentially fertile between Day 5 and Day 22. The fertile window remains the same whether you are aged 20 or 40.

Ovulating fewer than 10 days before the beginning of your next cycle could indicate that you have insufficient progesterone in your system or that you have imbalances in other hormones, such as FSH. Only a blood test will be able to tell you exactly when you've ovulated (see box, page 21), but your fertile indicators (see below) will give you a good idea of when ovulation is likely.

Your fertile indicators

You may have noticed that at certain times in your cycle you have an increased desire for sex – this is usually around your fertile time. Any abdominal pain or breast tenderness in the middle of your cycle may be good fertility indicators. Once you understand how your cycle works, you can also begin charting your temperature and making a note of your vaginal secretions to further guide you on when you are most likely to be fertile.

Temperature

Taking your temperature is only as reliable as your general health – taking medication, lack of sleep, and low-level illness can all affect your temperature. For this reason, I don't recommend that you rely completely upon temperature as a firm fertility indicator – although charting it over a few months can offer reassurance for when ovulation is likely to occur.

Chart your basal body temperature every day first thing on waking, before you get out of bed. Use a digital thermometer, which will give you a reading to tenths of a degree. Note down your temperature every day on a chart that begins on Day 1 of your cycle. On the morning immediately after you have ovulated, a surge in progesterone will cause a small temperature rise, which will then fall again to normal levels on subsequent days. Note that the temperature rise itself occurs after ovulation, so past your most fertile time.

Vaginal secretions

As oestrogen rises and your body prepares for ovulation, the cells of the cervix produce secretions that help the sperm move towards the egg. These fertile secretions are the best, natural indicator you have of your fertile time.

Day 1 of your cycle is the first day of your period, during which bleeding will typically last for between three and five days. Once bleeding stops, you may have some dry days with very little vaginal secretion at all. Then may come some creamy-white secretions. As you approach ovulation, these become thinner and wetter and increase in quantity. Just prior to ovulation they become clear and stretchy and are often described as resembling raw egg white. At this point you are thought to be at the peak time for your fertility. Almost immediately following ovulation, when progesterone rises, secretions stop and a seal into the cervix is formed to prevent any more sperm getting through.

Note that if you are older (say, in your late-thirties or early forties) you may have fewer secretions altogether. In addition, certain over-the-counter medications such as antihistamines will dry up vaginal secretions.

The diet plan and your cycle

Mood, weight and hormones can change rapidly according to where a woman is in her cycle. It is possible to support your body's monthly shifts through your diet. Furthermore, being in tune with your natural rhythms will help you stick to the EYP Fertility Diet plan.

We often hear the word 'regular' with reference to the ideal woman's cycle. Medically speaking regular is any cycle that varies in length by no more than seven days, month to month. If your cycle fluctuates more than this – for example, if it is 25 days long one month, 32 the next month and 42 the next – ovulation becomes hard to predict and your cycle is said to be irregular. It is likely that the unpredictability is the result of hormonal imbalances. The right nutrition at the right time of the month can make a big difference when it comes to getting your cycle into a healthier pattern.

The EYP Fertility Diet encourages you to eat the right foods for your time of the month. If you can do so, you should start to bring your hormones back into balance. This should make conception that crucial bit more likely.

Eating right for your cycle

In this section I want to encourage you to think about how you feel at each of the stages (phases) in your cycle. Then, I'll tell you which foods will help support your shifting moods and emotions (a natural by-product of your changing hormones) over the course of the month.

Phase one

Many women can actually feel the hormonal shift on the first day of their period – pent-up tension seems to fall away and a sense of relief and calm ensues. However, like many other women, you may also feel a bit depleted or lethargic. Take some time out when your period begins – enjoy some quiet time that allows you to conserve and then restore your energy. Avoid exercising and treat yourself to an early night (or two).

This is a time for warm, nourishing foods. Choose a diet rich in iron and vitamin C, as these nutrients help to replenish the iron that you lose with your period. Vitamin-B-rich foods will help you to regain some energy. Good sources of iron include lean red meat, pumpkin seeds, beans and pulses, dried apricots and raisins, shellfish and dark green leafy vegetables. For B-vitamins include whole grains, lamb, beef, poultry, shellfish, eggs, and dairy products, leafy green vegetables, yeast extract and nutritional yeast flakes. Most fruits and vegetables will provide good levels of vitamin C (this is essential for iron absorption), but particularly good sources of vitamin C include citrus fruits, berries, kiwi fruit, leafy green vegetables and red pepper.

If you suffer from period pain, try taking an omega-3 supplement to help reduce levels of inflammation in your body.

Phase two

During this phase, which can vary in length from month to month, oestrogen is on the rise as your body prepares for ovulation. Many women feel great – attractive, flirty, full of libido. This is usually a time when you'll burst with energy – you may feel like hitting the gym or pounding the streets (if that's your thing). Now is the time to notice some of the vital signs and secretions associated with this fertile time of the month (see page 25).

During this phase, stock up on your B-vitamins (see opposite), which are important for hormonal balance. B-vitamins also help with healthy cell division (a crucial part of babymaking). Lecithin (a phospholipid found in animal products) will help to keep your cell membranes healthy. Keep eating the vitamin-C-rich foods as this vitamin is thought to increase the amount of water in your cervical mucus, making it more plentiful. Foods rich in capsaicin, isoflavones and L-arginine (such as, in turn, spicy foods, tofu and watermelon) encourage the body to make nitric oxide (NO). This compound helps to dilate your blood vessels, easing blood flow through your whole system, which is good news for your reproductive organs (including your genitals, uterus and ovaries).

Finally, for healthy implantation to occur during this crucial part of your cycle, your immune system needs to be in optimum condition. For this reason, stock up on vitamin D – the workhorse of your immunity. Exposing your skin to sunlight is the best way to get your body to manufacture this vitamin, but it is also present in salmon and sardines, and in shiitake mushrooms (if you're vegetarian).

Phase three

This is the luteal phase of your cycle (see page 10). The corpus luteum (the ruptured ovarian follicle that produces progesterone to thicken the womb lining, close the cervix and maintain a pregnancy) contains a high level of betacarotene, which is the orange–yellow pigment found mainly in foods such as carrots and butternut squash, as well as other vegetables. Betacarotene is also a powerful antioxidant – a free-radical scavenger that helps protect your cells from damage. During this phase of your cycle, try to include plenty of betacarotene-rich foods in your diet, including butternut squash, carrots, collards, kale, spinach, sweet potato and mustard greens.

Phase four

If no fertilization has occurred, your hormone levels start to fall. During this phase you may begin to feel more lethargic again – it's this time (on the run-up to your period) that many women find they crave sweet foods. Remember your 80:20 leeway and allow yourself the odd treat, but try to make sure that generally you eat foods that will keep your blood sugar stable (slow-releasing carbs; see page 37). Your cycle begins again at the end of this phase – marked by the moment you get your period.

It takes two – the fatherhood factor

Despite the fact that conception takes place in the woman's body and that she will carry the baby, we now know that half of all fertility problems are down to what's going on inside the man. This means that the fertility diet is important for fathers-to-be, too.

In some ways men are luckier than women – whereas a woman is born with all the eggs she will ever have in her lifetime, a man will produce sperm 24 hours a day for seven days a week. While there comes a time in a woman's life when she is no longer able to become a mother, a man can become a father (in theory) until his dying day. Nonetheless, studies show that men shouldn't become complacent. Here, I want to focus on what's going on inside the man's body and show you why it's so important that fathers follow the fertility diet, too.

The structure of sperm

The sperm cell is much, much smaller than the egg cell and consists of the head (which contains the genetic material), the mid-piece (which is the energy powerhouse of the sperm) and the tail (which propels the sperm forward). The head of the sperm is covered with a cap called the acrosome, a fine membrane that is vulnerable to damage and has to come off before the sperm can penetrate the egg.

Making sperm

The most important role a man has in the process of babymaking is to deliver healthy DNA via sperm carried in his semen. Most of the fluid in semen is made up of secretions from the male reproductive organs and contains citric acid, amino acids, fructose, enzymes, prostaglandin, potassium and zinc. Semen is slightly alkaline.

Sperm are made in special tubules, called seminiferous tubules, in the testes. It takes around 100 days altogether for each sperm to become fully grown – 74 days for a single sperm to develop, before it moves from the tubules into a coiled tube called the epididymis, where it spends 20 to 30 days maturing. Over that time, what a man eats and the lifestyle choices he makes can have their own impact on how healthy each and every one of his sperm will be.

Sperm need enormous amounts of energy. Think of the scale of the journey they undertake relative to their size. From inside the scrotal sac, they are propelled out of the penis into the woman. Passing along the woman's reproductive tract to get to the egg is like a human swimming the Pacific Ocean. But each sperm not only has to make the journey, it also has to win the race. Each sperm swims as fast as it can to get to the woman's fallopian tube first. Once there, the

Do men have a monthly cycle?

We all know that women have a monthly hormone cycle that sees their fertility levels rise and fall over the course of around 30 days (give or take a few). What we rarely come across is the idea that men have a hormone cycle, too.

Men begin producing sex hormones only during puberty (which means they produce sperm only once puberty has begun; a woman has all her eggs from the moment she is born). At some point between the ages of 11 and 14 (rarely earlier, but sometimes later), the testes become mature enough to begin producing testosterone – the so-called male hormone (although, as we've seen, women have some testosterone, too). Once testosterone kicks in, it ensures a constantly replenished supply of sperm, every day.

The fact that men have a perpetual sperm supply has mostly led us to assume that there is no monthly ebb and flow of male hormones – that men are not hormonal over the course of the month in the way that women might be. But is this right? Frustratingly, there is no definitive answer. Some schools of thought claim that men do have a monthly cycle, but this notion is not yet scientifically accepted. Testosterone levels do peak and trough over the course of day, though – with the highest levels in the morning (when men often feel most desire; see page 12) and the lowest in the evening.

Without a monthly cycle as complex as the woman's, men lack some of the clearer signs – irregular periods and so on – that women have of a potential issue with their fertility.

winning sperm has to drill into the egg to download its most precious genetic material.

Forty million sperm or more are ejaculated and begin to make this journey. At ejaculation a large amount of seminal fluid is produced. Sixty-five per cent of it is made up of fructose to give the sperm energy for their journey. The remainder of the ejaculate comes from the prostate and is rich in zinc, which sperm need in order to stay healthy on their journey and to stabilize their DNA.

Despite the millions of sperm that enter the woman's body, only about 200 will reach the fallopian tube, helped by the woman's alkaline vaginal secretions. Sperm can usually survive between three and five days once inside the woman's body.

What is the sperm carrying?
The head of the sperm contains half a baby's DNA (half the baby's genetic blueprint; the other half is

in the woman's egg). In the egg, the DNA is tightly packed into an X sex chromosome. Sperm may carry their DNA in either an X or a Y sex chromosome. The sperm's chromosome pairs with the egg's chromosome to make either XX (which results in a baby girl) or XY (a boy).

What constitutes healthy sperm?

In each ejaculate there are millions of sperm but not all are normal – in fact, a high percentage is abnormal. To assess the health of the sperm, a doctor will make a semen analysis. This looks at the sperm count (the number of sperm per millilitre of semen), sperm motility (quality of motion) and sperm morphology (shape), assessing the head, tail and neck of the sperm.

Key factors for healthy reproduction are:

- the ejaculate needs to contain more than 20 million sperm per millilitre
- the volume of each ejaculate needs to be 2 millilitres
- more than 50 per cent of the sperm in each needs to be moving properly
- 4 per cent or more of the sperm need to have normal morphology. (Given that only 4 per cent morphology is considered normal, it is important that all the other parameters are good!)

We can see all these physical characteristics under a microscope, but what the microscope can't immediately show is whether within the sperm free radicals will have damaged the DNA.

What nutrients do healthy sperm need?

The health of the sperm begins with the health of the semen, which contains 22 different nutrients and is rich in minerals – notably calcium, magnesium, phosphorus and zinc, and vitamins B12 and C. Every man should ensure his diet provides a good intake of these vital nutrients.

Proteins contain amino acids that are essential building blocks for sperm (protein is also an excellent fuel source). Foods containing the amino acids L-arginine, L-carnitine and L-lysine are all important. Those rich in proteins including L-arginine are fish, poultry and red meat, and dairy products. Once in the body, this amino acid helps to produce nitric oxide (NO), which dilates blood vessels and improves circulation. Better circulation to the groin boosts sperm health and increases sperm motility. L-arginine also plays an important role in cell division, immune function and the release of hormones, and good levels may even improve sperm count.

Folic acid (a B-vitamin found, for example, in broccoli, Brussels sprouts, peas and chickpeas) is just as important for men as it is for women because it protects the sperm from DNA damage, including having too many or too few chromosomes (known as aneuploidy).

A number of nutrients help to improve the quality of sperm. Vitamin D may boost motility, while zinc improves the quality of the seminal fluid, and increases sperm count, motility and fertilizing capacity, and decreases levels of DNA damage, structural abnormalities and antibodies to sperm that can impair sperm quality.

Lifestyle and free-radical damage

Although sperm actually need low levels of free radicals in order to function (and this is why free radicals are generated naturally as the sperm make their way to the fallopian tubes), higher levels will damage the sperm cells.

In order to give the sperm the best possible chances of being strong enough and having enough energy to make their journey into the fallopian tube – and of fertilizing an egg successfully when they get there – avoiding excess oxidative stress as much as possible is essential.

Causes of free-radical damage in men
- heat – jacuzzis, tight underwear, heated car seats, mobile phones in pockets and laptops on laps all raise the temperature of the testes, which hang outside the body for the very reason that sperm are damaged by heat!
- charred barbecued foods
- trans fats (such as those found in processed foods, deep-fried foods and takeaways)
- alcohol, nicotine (smoking) and other recreational drugs
- age, but a healthy diet and lifestyle will keep all the body systems younger for longer

In order to provide sperm with all the energy they need to make their epic journey, men need a good intake of L-carnitine. This amino acid carries high-energy fat compounds into mitochondria cells, where they are burned to release their energy. (Vegans should be aware that plant foods contain no L-carnitine, so must supplement.)

Co-enzyme Q10 is another important nutrient for the conversion of food to energy in the cells. It is also boosts sperm motility, because the mid-piece of the sperm needs this nutrient specifically to get the sperm moving and sustain energy to the tail to drive the sperm onwards.

Omega-3 fatty acids (see pages 34–5) are essential for sperm health for several reasons.

They give the sperm flexibility, helping the head to penetrate the egg. In addition, sperm cells must have specific membrane characteristics in order to be able to bind to the membrane of an egg and produce a living embryo. Much of those special characteristics come from the sperm's high levels of omega-3 fatty acids.

Men with poor sperm quality or sperm counts may typically have low levels of omega-3s, or low ratios of omega-3 to omega-6 fats in their semen and sperm-cell composition. Studies indicate that supplementation with omega-3s can improve total sperm count and concentration. One study showed that an omega-3-rich Mediterranean-style diet boosted the chances of successful pregnancy in previously infertile couples by a staggering 40 per cent. Finally, antioxidants are a must – a good intake protects the health of the head of the sperm (which contains the DNA).

What damages sperm?

Apart from sexually transmitted infections, such as chlamydia (which can damage the tubules in which sperm are made and therefore damage sperm) and heat, there is now much evidence that free radicals can damage the DNA that lies within the sperm head. In fact, studies show that at least 30 to 80 per cent of male infertility is linked to oxidative stress (free-radical damage). It appears that these marauding free-radical cells damage the fatty layers of membranes, such as the acrosome that covers the sperm's genetic material. (It's now possible to test for DNA fragmentation – which indicates the likelihood of DNA damage to sperm.)

However, oxidative stress is a natural by-product of generating all the energy sperm need to make it to the fallopian tube. And it's not only the DNA that can be affected. Free radicals damage all the sperm cell membranes and the mitochondria (that convert food energy into usable energy), too. Studies show that men with elevated markers of oxidation have generally impaired sperm count and more abnormally formed cells.

No matter where in the body free-radical damage has occurred, including inside the sperm, the best treatment is quite simply to boost the levels of antioxidants in your diet. Those with

more antioxidants in their diet have higher sperm counts and better motility. A number of specific antioxidants have proven ability to boost sperm quality. These include vitamins C and E (which help to prevent the sperm clumping, giving them better motility and improving the health of sperm membranes respectively), co-enzyme Q10, selenium (especially for healthy sperm formation and motility), n-acetylcysteine (NAC) and zinc. Lycopene is a natural, plant-derived carotenoid pigment that provides the red colour of tomatoes, watermelon and other fruits. It has powerful antioxidant characteristics. Studies have shown that a lycopene supplement can improve sperm concentration and motility and the general health of the sperm.

The diet for fathers

The EYP Fertility Diet is one of the most powerful health changes that any father-to-be can make to ensure that he produces the best possible sperm with the best possible chances of making a baby. Because numerous studies show that specific changes to diet can increase the chances of healthy ovulation and producing a healthy embryo, prevent recurrent miscarriage and support a healthy pregnancy, there are many diets intended only for the woman. This diet provides all the essential nutrients to support healthy egg production, but it also gives you everything you need for healthy sperm production, too. Both men and women will benefit from all the hormone-balancing nutrients in the diet. It bursts with antioxidants that will

Key antioxidants and their food sources

This list is one of the most important you will ever read for your health. The following foods are antioxidant superstars and should feature in your diet as often as possible. Keep the list somewhere where you can both see it – because it is important for both of you.

Vitamin C Berries, citrus fruits; leafy green vegetables, red peppers

Vitamin E Nuts and seeds and their oils

Co-enzyme Q10 Beef, chicken, pork; salmon, trout; broccoli; oranges

Selenium Lamb, turkey; cod, halibut, salmon, sardines, tuna; Brazil nuts

N-acetylcysteine Chicken, duck, pork, turkey; dairy, eggs; broccoli, onions, red peppers

Lycopene Guava, grapefruit, Sharon fruit, tomatoes, watermelon

Zinc Beef, chicken, lamb, pork; spinach; oysters; pumpkin seeds, nuts, wheatgerm; cocoa

help to protect the sperm from free radicals, and with cell-energizing nutrients that will optimize the chances of the sperm making it into the fallopian tube.

Remember that hormone balance also requires reducing stress levels – and stress affects a man's fertility (and particularly libido) as much as it affects a woman's. I encourage men to read the section on lifestyle (see pages 51–5).

Finally, I think it's very important that men feel involved in the process of making a baby. So often I see couples and it is the woman whose anxiety has brought them to me, while the man feels inhibited and exposed by the process. Reading this book together,

undertaking the principles together – from the diet changes to the lifestyle ideas – will help you stay connected. And that is just as important as any of the other advice I've given in the book.

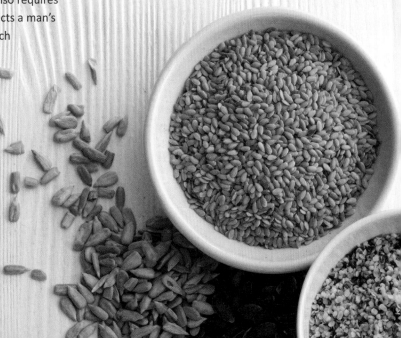

Getting your body baby-ready – diet

Now that you know about how your fertility works, we need to get down to the nitty gritty of making sure you do everything you can to get your body baby-ready. This begins with ensuring that your diet provides all the nutrients you need for optimal hormonal balance.

The latest national diet and nutrition surveys in the UK and USA reveal a worrying trend. They show that we have insufficient intake of key nutrients such as vitamin D, folic acid, iron, magnesium and omega-3 fats, and that we increasingly rely upon processed convenience foods rather than on fresh, whole foods. Furthermore, even if we do eat a healthy diet, modern methods of production and storage mean that the nutrient content of our food is often lower than the levels of 50 years ago. To make matters worse, stress and environmental toxins further deplete the nutrients in our bodies. For optimal fertility, we need to redress the balance.

The power of protein

It's not only your hormones and the neurotransmitters in your brain that need protein – eggs and sperm need it, too. High-quality protein, such as from lean meat and poultry, as well as fish, eggs and soya beans, contains all eight essential amino acids. These are biological catalysts that enable protein to break down and become what the body needs – be that muscle or other tissue, egg, sperm, neurotransmitter or hormone. Your body can't manufacture these

amino acids for itself (which is why they are essential), so they must come from your diet. Include one portion (about the size of your fist) of protein in every meal. If you're vegetarian or vegan, you'll need a full range of plant proteins to ensure that you get all the essential amino acids (see box, opposite).

Fat facts

Women tend to need more fat than men for the healthy production of hormones. Healthy fats, such as those found in oily fish and certain seeds, stimulate the action of beneficial prostaglandins within the body. These are fat cells that play a critical role in menstruation, conception, pregnancy and labour. Unhealthy fats, such as saturated fats and trans fats, are quite simply villains who hamper fertility!

Essential fatty acids (EFAs)

Healthy fats that your body can't produce for itself, EFAs must come from your diet. There are several kinds, but the most important for fertility and conception are omega-3 fats. Not only are these crucial for hormone production, they also help to modulate the immune system, reduce

The vegetarian and vegan fertility diet

As protein is such a key element of the fertility diet (to make healthy eggs), it's important to know what sources there are for vegans and vegetarians. Beans, leafy greens, pulses, nuts and seeds are all good vegan sources, while vegetarians can add in eggs and dairy foods, too. I'd also encourage you to use protein powders – including hemp, pea and sprouted-seed-based powders.

Finally, be aware that vegetarians and vegans may be more prone to other nutritional deficiencies that can affect fertility – including low levels of iodine, iron, omega-3 fatty acids, vitamin B12 and vitamin D. Supplement with a multivitamin and -mineral formula to make sure that you keep all your vitamin and mineral levels up, and vegans may also need to take a specific vitamin B12 supplement, too.

inflammation and boost mood. Omega-3 fats help to balance compounds in the body known as eicosanoids, which may be linked to increased risk of miscarriage. Studies of pregnant women who consume large amounts of long-chain omega-3 fatty acids, such as EPA (eicosapentaenoic acid) and DHA (docosahexaenoic acid), both of which are found in fish oil, tend to carry their babies for longer and have a correspondingly lower rate of premature birth.

Monounsaturated fats

This healthy type of fat can have a beneficial effect on insulin levels, helping to stabilize blood sugar, which has positive effects for your fertility. Monounsaturated fats remain liquid at room temperature, so are found in healthy oils, such as olive oil and sesame oil, and in nuts and seeds.

Saturated fats

Typically found in animal and dairy products, saturated fats, when eaten to excess, can interfere with your cell membranes (including those involved in reproduction). Furthermore, they may directly affect a man's fertility by reducing the quality and quantity of his sperm. Saturated fats that contain medium-chain triglycerides (MCTs) – such as coconut oil – are more stable than other types of saturated fat, making them comparatively more healthy. These are more readily broken down by the liver and your body can use them for energy production.

Trans fats

Found in processed or fried foods and some margarines, trans fats (also known as damaged, hydrogenated or partially hydrogenated fats) prevent your body from making good use of

Full-fat is good for fertility

Many women make the mistake of substituting foods containing fat with low-fat products, thinking they won't gain weight using them. However, for fertility – and, for that matter, for weight management – the principle is flawed. These products often contain trans fats, sugar and sweeteners. Artificial sweeteners disrupt the normal hormonal and neurological signals that control hunger and satiety. Many studies have shown that a diet that is high in sweeteners in the end leads to a greater consumption of calories and so to weight gain.

But, weight aside, there is some startling evidence for how low-fat products can hamper conception. In one extensive study in the USA, women who ate two or more low-fat dairy products a day were twice as likely to have problems conceiving. Ovulation rates were 38 per cent better among those who used full-fat milk. One reason for this might be that when the fat is skimmed off dairy products to make reduced-fat versions, oestrogen and progesterone are removed, too, leaving an unnatural preponderance of androgens (male hormones).

essential fats and are generally harmful for all aspects of health, including fertility. All processed oils contain trans fats and they regularly appear in foods marketed as low fat (see box, above).

How much and what kind?

Fats should comprise around 30 per cent of your diet, but no more than 10 per cent should come from saturated fats, and you should avoid trans fats altogether. The fats in your fertility diet should come from foods rich in EFAs and monounsaturated fats. This works out at a maximum intake of approximately 70g (2½oz) of fat per day for women and 95g (3¼oz) per day for men. As a guide to what this means in practice,

one avocado contains almost 30g (1oz) of fat, a tablespoon of olive oil contains 14g (½oz) fat.

Monounsaturated fats include olive oil, rapeseed oil and rice bran oil, as well as the natural oils in avocados, most nuts and seeds, and organic, free-range poultry.

Omega-3-rich foods include oily fish (such as mackerel, salmon and sardines), rapeseed oil, linseeds (flaxseeds), chia, hemp and pumpkin seeds, and walnuts. Another type of essential fat, omega-6, occurs in raw seeds, especially chia, hemp, pumpkin, sesame and sunflower seeds, and their oils.

Carbohydrates

Your body needs carbohydrate for energy, but the quality of those carbs is critical. Good carbs are known as complex. These are slowly broken down into glucose (which the body uses as fuel), and are steadily released into the blood stream. You may hear them referred to as low-glycaemic-load (GL) carbohydrates. Because low-GL carbs are more nutritionally dense than other kinds, they help to keep your blood-sugar levels stable. Beans, pulses, vegetables, whole grains and some fruits, such as berries and citrus fruits, are all good sources. And if you combine good protein, good fats and good carbohydrates at each meal, you'll be doing the best you can to balance your blood sugar. Eliminate refined sugars, sodas, processed fruit juices and artificial sweeteners – as these are all sources of bad carbohydrate that release sugar into the blood stream too quickly, causing insulin imbalance.

Antioxidants

During metabolism, your body produces free radicals – unstable molecules that race through you trying to make themselves more stable. In doing this, they damage otherwise healthy cells. Toxins, pollution and a poor lifestyle (including smoking and getting sunburnt) can also cause free-radical damage (also known as oxidative stress) within the body. Male infertility, endometriosis and damage to egg cells and to sperm have all been linked with the action of free radicals. Wonderfully, there are brave warriors against free-radical damage – antioxidants.

There are two types of antioxidant – endogenous antioxidants that are made by the body, and exogenous that you obtain from your diet and supplements. Fruit and vegetables are packed with powerful phytonutrients (plant nutrients) that are potent antioxidants. Think colour – the darker or brighter the colour of the fruit or vegetable, the greater its antioxidant power. Nuts and seeds, herbs, spices (particularly turmeric) and green tea are also good sources. See the box on page 33 for some more ideas.

Reality check

So, your baby-ready diet needs to be perfectly balanced with good protein, good fats, good carbs and an abundance of antioxidants. No more will you look at chocolate bars and fizzy drinks; crisps and cakes are for the old you... Well, yes in a perfect world. But I don't want you to be perfect; I want you to be realistic. For many women (in particular), food, mood and hormones are interlinked. You might crave different foods at different times in your cycle. It's possible to tailor your diet to take into account the ebb and flow of your cycle, so that you can eat more healthily when your hormones allow, and leave yourself a little bit of leeway for the times when nothing but chocolate will do. Take a look at pages 26–7 for some tips on how to eat in tune with your cycle.

Overall, I recommended an 80:20 approach – try to stick to my recommendations 80 per cent of the time and don't worry if you occasionally slip up (that is, you have a 20-per cent leeway).

The need for detox

I want to give you a clean-slate position from which to start preparing for pregnancy. So, before you embark upon applying the principles of the baby-ready diet, it's important you try a detox (intended for both of you) that you'll find straightforward to implement and will help get your body back to basics. Don't panic! I've created one that's only five days long (see pages 42–4)! The body's natural detoxing organ is the liver, and the aim of the detox programme is to reduce the burden on it, which (as you've seen) will help balance your oestrogen levels and help you to kick any bad habits.

Having prepared with your detox, there are certain general principles that I want to encourage you to adopt in your diet over the coming months. These are to get your gut healthy and your blood sugar in balance, and to create a less acidic environment in your body, which is not only better for you generally, but a better environment for sperm.

Loving your gut – fertility and digestion

As you've seen, your hormones are made by the nutrients in your system. This means that your gut needs to be in super condition to get the best out of your food. Here are my top tips for gut health.

1. Eat the right foods

The Chinese believe that foods have five flavours – sweet, sour, salty, bitter and fragrant. All are thought to create different energies in the body, which affect the flow of *qi* (the body's life force).

In order to be healthy, the Chinese believe we need a balance of all these flavours in our diet. Whether or not you hold with the Chinese view, the notion of balance is one that is crucially important for good gut health. Try to implement the 80:20 approach to eating (see page 37) and make sure you get a range of nutrients.

2. Eat at the right times

Your digestion is raring to go at breakfast. This is why having a good breakfast that includes slow-releasing carbohydrates is essential at the start of the day. Breakfast is the most important time to set yourself up to avoid snacking. I'm not a great one for snacks – I think that if you eat good carbs, you shouldn't feel the need to snack between mealtimes. Take your main meal at lunchtime twice or three times a week if you can. This avoids a heavy meal in the evening, which may interfere with your digestion. (Focus more on protein and vegetables – and less on carbs – in your evening meals, as these are less taxing for your gut. Carbs, raw foods and alcohol after 7pm can result in a combination of sugars that ferment in your gut, causing gas and acidity that weaken your gut lining.) Also, a late supper means that you're taking in a lot of fuel, but not doing anything with it, so it is stored as fat. Finally, but importantly, if your body is busy trying to digest food at night, you won't be able to sleep properly.

3. Eat the right amount

Increasingly, the Western population in particular is overeating. As a guide, don't eat until you can't

Immunity and fertility

In order to accept the sperm, and so the embryo, your immune system has to be in optimal condition. Between 70 and 75 per cent of your immune cells reside in your gut, which means that gut health is essential for immunity, but also (looking at it the other way) that a gut-friendly diet helps to boost your immunity.

Poor lifestyle and poor nutrition will over time weaken your immunity, but there are plenty of foods that can help to build it up.

Top immunity-boosting foods
Apples, berries, betacarotene-rich foods (such as butternut squash, carrot, pumpkin, sweet potato), cherries, eggs, garlic, ginger, probiotics (including fermented foods such as kefir, live yogurt, miso, natto, sauerkraut and tempeh), mushrooms (particularly shiitake mushrooms), nuts and seeds (which are rich in the antioxidants vitamin E, zinc and selenium), oats, oily fish, onion, turmeric, super-green powders, and whey protein powder.

take any more – stop before you get full. Use a smaller plate so that what's on it looks lavish rather than mean; and savour every mouthful to fully appreciate what you're eating.

4. Chew, chew, chew
As a child weren't you always told to chew properly? Chewing is the first stage of the digestion process, increasing the salivary enzymes that help to break down your food before it gets to your stomach, making it easier to digest. By chewing your food you also feel fuller for longer and so are less likely to snack or overeat.

No more rollercoaster – blood-sugar balance
In order to make sure your blood-sugar levels remain stable, follow these simple principles:

• Don't skip meals.
• Combine protein and carbohydrate at every meal. This delays the digestive process and allows a more gradual release of glucose into your blood stream. You will feel fuller for longer and are less likely to have an energy dip that makes you want to snack on something sweet. Peas and beans are a ready-made mixture of protein and carbohydrate, so stock up on them.
• Avoid refined carbohydrates and processed foods – including sugary cakes, biscuits and sweets, juice drinks or squashes, white bread and white rice and pasta. These are bad carbohydrates that release sugar too quickly into your blood stream and put you back on that rollercoaster of energy highs and lows.

How to reduce inflammation

Inflammation is your body's natural response to injury or illness. However, chronic (prolonged) inflammation can lead to insulin resistance and studies suggest it is linked to many conditions that may affect fertility, such as endometriosis, PCOS, implantation failure and recurrent miscarriage. Processed sugar and refined carbohydrates, and trans fats, as well as food allergies, infections, environmental toxins, stress and obesity can all trigger an inflammatory response in the body. To reduce inflammation you need to eliminate the underlying causes, and include plenty of anti-inflammatory foods in your diet every day.

Top dietary anti-inflammatories

Aloe vera, apples, bee propolis, berries, boswellia, buckwheat, chia seeds, devil's claw, garlic, ginger, grapeseed extract, green tea, hemp seed, liquorice, linseed (flaxseed), oily fish, olive oil, onion, papaya, pineapple, probiotics, rosemary, super-green powders, turmeric and walnuts.

- Eat slow-releasing low-GL carbohydrates – brown, dense and grainy foods that have all the vitamins, minerals and fibre still retained.
- Add a little unsaturated fat to your meals – almonds, avocado, olives, peanuts, pine nuts and sunflower seeds, and cold-pressed organic olive oil are all good sources.
- Always read the label. If sugar is one of the first ingredients listed (even if it's as organic cane juice, honey, agave, maple syrup, molasses or fructose syrup), put the product back.
- Snack between meals only if you are really hungry. If you must have something, make sure it's the right kind of snack. Nuts and seeds; oat cakes with hummus, cottage cheese, guacamole or nut butter; or fresh fruit with a spoonful of live yogurt are all examples of good-for-you snacks.

Acid–alkaline balance

Sperm thrive in a slightly alkaline environment. This is why vaginal secretions during a woman's fertile time are slightly alkaline. The pH of your blood is around 7.35–7.45, which is also slightly alkaline. Keeping your diet more alkaline is easier on your digestive system and will help your body maintain its natural acid–alkaline balance.

Although the body prefers to be slightly alkaline, acidity is a normal by-product of your metabolism. Acids are created when your body converts fats, proteins and carbohydrates into energy; then, they are excreted as waste.

High-protein diets, high alcohol intake and eating processed foods, as well as stress and smoking, all make the body more acidic.

In order to maintain acid–alkaline balance, 80 per cent of your food intake should be alkaline – which means eating plenty of alkaline-rich vegetables and some fruit with each meal. Use the following lists as a guide to the acidic (or otherwise) nature of certain foods. Try not to become too fixated on them, though – just be aware. As long as your diet is varied and healthy, your body should sort out the rest.

Alkaline-forming foods (include these):
- most fruits
- fresh vegetables and sea vegetables
- apple cider vinegar
- coconut water
- super-green powders, such as spirulina
- oils, such as avocado, olive, coconut and flaxseed

Neutral foods (include these):
- most nuts and seeds
- beans and pulses
- rice, soya and hemp protein powders
- buckwheat, chia, quinoa, lentils and tofu

Acid-forming foods (keep to a minimum):
- animal protein (meat, fish and so on)
- processed grains and cereals
- dairy products and eggs
- dried fruits, except dried figs
- sugar
- salt
- trans fats
- alcohol, caffeine, energy drinks and sodas

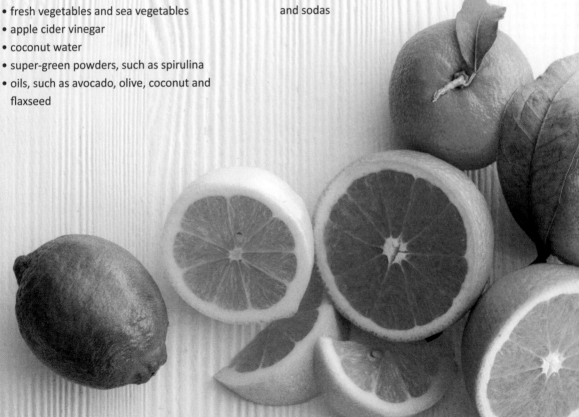

The EYP five-day fertility detox

Before embarking upon the EYP Fertility Diet, I recommend that you follow a five-day fertility cleanse. The cleanse will support your body's natural detoxification processes by providing nutrient-dense foods and drinks that support the liver in its role as your body's detoxifier.

Every day your body produces an array of compounds and internal waste products that it needs to dispose of safely. The food, drink and medications you consume, hidden environmental chemicals in bodycare and household products, electromagnetic radiation and environmental pollutants all add to this toxic load, placing a burden on your liver and its detox supporters – your kidneys and digestive system.

The five-day detox is intended for both of you to do together. Exposure to environmental toxins has been shown to affect male and female fertility. Many environmental toxins are endocrine disruptors, which means they interfere with your body's hormones, potentially resulting in decreased sperm quality, disrupted reproductive cycles and ovarian dysfunction.

Preparing for your fertility detox

The first stage of the cleanse is to remove all foods and toxins that may be placing additional burden on your digestive system and liver function. I suggest you cut out all alcohol, sugar and caffeine from your diet two or three days before you begin. If you don't already eat organic,

switching to organic produce can also help reduce your toxic load.

Plan your detox for days when you have sufficient time to rest and can avoid social functions, meals out and parties. If you can, schedule in some time every day to undertake gentle exercise such as swimming, Pilates, yoga or walking. Some people prefer to follow the plan around a weekend – I recommend beginning on a Thursday – but others like to complete it during the week. Choose what works best for you.

For the first two days you will eat three meals with the option of a healthy snack to eat mid-morning or mid-afternoon if you are really hungry. It is important to keep your blood-sugar levels balanced throughout the detox to avoid placing additional pressure on your adrenal glands. For this reason the cleanse includes protein-rich foods.

The following two days comprise a liquid-only diet with a range of smoothies, soups and juices throughout the day. Then, you complete the detox with a further day of three light meals and optional snacks. In order to support detoxification it is important to maintain the right acid–alkaline balance (see pages 40–1). The detox foods include lots of ingredients that support and maintain your body's natural alkalinity.

Allocate time to shop for all the ingredients before you begin and follow the meal planner every day.

Drink plenty of fluids – aim for 1 litre (35fl oz) of filtered water daily and also include a variety of herbal teas. Each day of the detox starts with a glass of hot water with a little lemon or lime juice added. This combination is very alkalizing and supports liver cleansing. You can also try adding ½ teaspoon of super-green powders to juices and smoothies daily.

Finishing the detox
At the end of Day 5 you should feel lighter, clearer and much more energized. Capitalize on your good work and immediately begin using the recipes in the rest of the book so that you don't have time to slip back into any bad habits. You are now on a path to a baby-ready body!

The inevitable don'ts
Try to steer clear of the following as they will hinder your attempts to detoxify:
- red meat, dairy foods, eggs, gluten grains (rye, barley and wheat), large fish (tuna, marlin, shark and swordfish) and shellfish
- sugary foods, charred foods, processed foods, deep-fried foods and foods high in trans fats and hydrogenated fats, and takeaways
- any foods wrapped in cling film or tin foil
- non-stick, aluminium or stainless steel cookware
- smoking or any recreational drugs

Detox-boosting supplements

Support your cleanse with an antioxidant supplement formula that includes many of the following nutrients. Talk to your local healthfood shop or pharmacy – someone there should be able to advise you on the best formula for you, based on a combination of these ingredients:
- glutathione and/or n-acetylcysteine (NAC)
- betacarotene
- B-vitamins, particularly B6, B12 and folic acid
- vitamin C
- vitamin E
- selenium
- omega-3 fats
- co-enzyme Q10
- alpha lipoic acid
- milk thistle (a herb that supports liver function)
- turmeric
- MSM (methyl-sulfonyl-methane)

The EYP fertility detox – day by day

DAY 1

On waking Start the day with a glass of warm water with a little added lemon juice, and drink slowly.

Breakfast The Deep Green Cleanse (p.58); Super Berry Chia Pudding (p.65)

Lunch Avocado, Orange & Sea Vegetable Salad with Sprouted Seeds (p.92)

Snack Wasabi Guacamole (p.100) with carrot sticks

Dinner Chilli-Glazed Salmon with Cucumber Lime Salad (p.124)

DAY 2

On waking Start the day with a glass of warm water with a little added lemon juice, and drink slowly.

Breakfast B Booster (p.59); Fruit & Mango Cream Parfait (p.62)

Lunch Flaked Trout with Rocket, Lychees & Sweet Lime Dressing (p.89)

Snack Mixed Seed Crackers (p.101) with Roasted Aubergine & Mint Dip (p.99)

Dinner Spinach, Walnut & Roasted Pear Salad with Raspberry Vinaigrette (p.91)

DAY 3 (LIQUID DAY)

On waking Start the day with a glass of warm water with a little added lemon juice, and drink slowly.

Breakfast Green Energizer (p.58)

Mid-morning Stress-Busting Mocha (p.61)

Lunch Roasted Butternut Squash & Ginger Soup with Hemp Pesto (p.79)

Mid-afternoon Avocado Antioxidant Fruit Blend (p.59)

Dinner Chunky Minestrone Soup (p.80)

Evening Strawberry Kefir (p.61)

DAY 4 (LIQUID DAY)

On waking Start the day with a glass of warm water with a little added lemon juice, and drink slowly.

Breakfast Stress-Busting Mocha (p.61)

Mid-morning The Deep Green Cleanse (p.58)

Lunch Chunky Minestrone Soup (p.80)

Mid-afternoon B Booster (p.59)

Dinner Broccoli, Fennel & Pear Soup (p.82)

Evening Avocado Antioxidant Fruit Blend (p.59)

DAY 5

On waking Start the day with a glass of warm water with a little added lemon juice, and drink slowly.

Breakfast The Deep Green Cleanse (p.58); Protein Boost Seeded Granola (p.68) with nut milk

Lunch Sicilian Quinoa Bowl (p.95)

Snack Tangy Tomato Kale Crisps (p.102)

Dinner Indonesian Chicken with Buckwheat Noodles (p.114)

How to choose, cook and store food

As well as making sure that what's on your plate is as colourful (colour means variety) and as unprocessed as possible, you'll need to follow a few simple guidelines to make certain that your body derives the most benefit it can from what you put into it. Try to eat as much organic produce as possible, but particularly aim for organic meat and dairy, and try to eat foods that have been produced locally so that they haven't lost nutrients during transportation.

When you're cooking, use cast iron, ceramic or glass, and avoid non-stick and aluminium cookware. Food, especially acidic foods such as citrus juices, can react with the coating or metal during the heating process and absorb some of the metal or coating toxins.

Cook at low temperatures as much as your recipes allow to prevent the creation of free radicals. Bake, boil, steam or stir-fry, and avoid using the microwave and frying with polyunsaturated oils. Use either a filter jug or a water filter built into your tap to purify water before you use it for cooking (or drinking). This will minimize your exposure to oestrogens and toxins in your water supply.

Avoid plastic food wraps. Research suggests that a compound in plastics known as bisphenol has been linked to male and female fertility issues. (Avoid plastic-wrapped sandwiches and ready meals, and plastic water bottles, for these reasons, too.) Do not heat food in plastic containers or put hot food in plastic containers to cool down (let it cool in a ceramic bowl first).

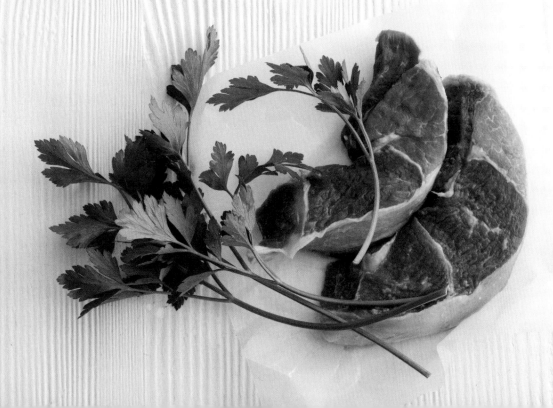

The EYP fertility diet

Good nutrition is the foundation of the Eat Yourself Pregnant programme. Now that you know how fertility works and the general principles of how to eat, you need to start implementing the EYP Fertility Diet. Remember it's for both you and your partner.

Much of the advice that follows has already come up in the discussions about how fertility works. Nonetheless, this is your one-stop-shop for the general principles you should follow when you do your food shopping. Then, with a little bit of luck and good timing, the rest will follow naturally.

Eat natural, whole foods

First things first – the quality of your food is paramount. Nutrient-dense foods both nourish and satisfy you. Keep processed foods to a minimum. Base your diet around fresh vegetables, sea vegetables, nuts and seeds, fermented foods such as yogurt and kefir, beans, pulses and, if you eat animal products, include free-range eggs, wild-caught fish, game and naturally reared animals. Ideally switch to organic.

Eat low-GL carbs

Slow-releasing carbohydrates avoid insulin spikes. Pile your plate full of vegetables; limit fruit to two portions a day; and consume between one and two portions of whole grains daily. Avoid white refined carbohydrates, processed foods and sugars.

Focus on alkalizing foods

A more alkaline diet is easier on your digestive system and will help your body maintain an acid–alkaline balance. Include plenty of alkalizing vegetables such as leafy green vegetables with each meal.

Avoid low-fat foods

Healthy fats and cholesterol are vital for your body, enabling the absorption of key nutrients and the production of hormones. Egg and sperm health depend upon an adequate supply of omega-3 fatty acids from oily fish and seeds. Include healthy saturated fats such as coconut oil, wild-caught fish, grass-fed meats and organic dairy and eggs, as well as monounsaturated fats such as those in extra virgin olive oil, nuts and avocados. Choose full-fat dairy foods rather than skimmed or semi-skimmed.

Eat your antioxidants

Aim to include a minimum of three portions of vegetables daily and two portions of fruit. See the box on page 33 for a list of key antioxidant foods that should become staples in your diet.

Include gut-friendly foods

Probiotics or healthy bacteria are essential for gut health and immunity. Eat fermented or cultured foods daily – including natural yogurt, kefir, sauerkraut, kimchi, miso, and pickled vegetables.

Plan your plate

How do you fill your plate? Aim to fill half of your plate with low-carb colourful vegetables; one-quarter with good-quality protein-rich foods (fish, seafood, meat, eggs, nuts, beans, lentils); and the remaining quarter with some starchy vegetables, such as potato or sweet potato, or whole grains (for example, rice or quinoa).

Drink plenty

Water is essential for digestion, nutrient absorption and transportation, cell health and the removal of toxins via the liver and kidneys. Keeping hydrated will promote energy levels and clear thinking. Aim for eight glasses of water or water-based liquid daily. Herbal teas, green juices and smoothies will contribute to this target; caffeine and carbonated drinks will not.

The EYP Fertility Diet recipes

The recipes on pages 58–157 have been developed to provide you with all the essential nutrients for fertility. Many of the recipes are quick and easy to prepare and can be made in advance. Take a look at the example food plan (illustrating just two days) below to give you a good understanding of how to balance your meals. You can then mix and match recipes and daily menus to suit your needs and tastes.

DAY	Breakfast	Lunch	Dinner	Snacks (optional)
1	Overnight Muesli (see p.67) with natural yogurt and a handful of berries	Chunky Minestrone Soup (p.80) Mixed Seed Crackers (p.101)	Roast Beef Fillet with Roasted Garlic, Tomato & Herb Sauce (p.123) and steamed vegetables	B Booster (p.59) Wasabi Guacamole (p.100) with vegetable sticks
2	Stress-Busting Mocha (p.61) 2 oat cakes with smoked salmon and cream cheese	Lebanese Fattoush Salad with Sumac-Roasted Chicken (p.83)	Moroccan-Spiced Mackerel (p.129) with steamed vegetables	Green Energizer (p.58) Tangy Tomato Kale Crisps (p.102)

Getting your body baby-ready – supplements

In an ideal world, we would derive all the nutrients we need from the food that we eat and the lifestyle we live. However, as this ideal becomes increasingly difficult to attain, I think that supplements should form an essential part of any fertility plan.

The Western population shows an increasing trend towards large-scale deficiencies in iron, folic acid and magnesium; omega-3 fats; and vitamin D. There are two main reasons why. First, modern farming and processing techniques deplete food of essential nutrients. Second, modern lifestyles expose us to more toxins and chronic stress, and keep us indoors and away from natural sunlight (which we need to manufacture vitamin D). The net result is that many of us need to take supplements to put our bodies back in balance.

Basic supplement plan
As a baseline, I recommend that both you and your partner supplement with a quality multivitamin and -mineral formula, which studies show can increase your chances of conceiving. I also recommend daily supplements of omega-3 fats (EPA and DHA) and perhaps of vitamin D and of folic acid. I also think most people will benefit from a high-quality probiotic, as well as perhaps an iodine supplement (ask your nutritionist to check your iodine levels first). Use the following to guide you when choosing your products.

Multivitamin and -mineral formula
As well as all the main vitamins and minerals, this formula should include antioxidants such as vitamins C and E, and the minerals selenium and zinc. Ideally, it should contain at least 100 per cent of the RDV (recommended daily value) of all the main vitamins and minerals. It is available in capsules and in powdered form.

Vitamin D
Also called the sunshine vitamin, vitamin D is manufactured in your skin when you expose it to ultraviolet light. Although there are important reasons why you should use sunblock, not allowing any part of the skin to be exposed to sunlight at any time does diminish your ability to make vitamin D. In the clinic we find that almost every person we test shows some level of vitamin-D deficiency. Black and Asian men and women tend to be particularly depleted, as are those who suffer from PCOS, are overweight or have coeliac disease. Spend 10 minutes every day out in the open air with sun on your face, but avoid the hours when the sun is at its hottest.

Myo-inositol – super-supplement

Inositol is a term used to refer to a group of naturally occurring carbohydrate compounds that exist in various forms. The most common is myo-inositol. Often sold as a dietary supplement, it can improve insulin sensitivity and it is thought to have many benefits for hormone balance and overcoming reproductive problems. Some studies show that deficiency in this compound is linked to PCOS (see page 22) and that supplementation can help even out otherwise irregular cycles and perhaps even improve egg quality. Talk to your nutritionist about adding this supplement to your pre-pregnancy supplementation plan.

Vitamin D supports the immune system and helps build healthy bone and muscle mass. It can improve blood-sugar balance and libido. Some IVF studies showed that women with higher levels in their follicular fluid were more likely to fall pregnant. For the man, higher levels of vitamin D means better sperm motility.

Check the levels of vitamin D in your daily multivitamin and -mineral and then consult a nutritionist or doctor and ask for a blood test to determine whether or not you could take a further vitamin-D supplement. Ideally blood levels should read between 60 and 80nmol/l. At high levels vitamin D is toxic to your body, so don't be tempted to supplement if you don't need to.

If your blood levels show that you do need a boost, ensure you take your supplement in the right form. Look for vitamin D3 cholecalciferol, not D2. After supplementing with vitamin D for between two and three months, ask for a further blood test to see if you should continue.

Omega-3 fatty acids (EPA and DHA)

Vital for cell membrane health, lowering inflammation and promoting good prostaglandins, omega-3 fatty acids also improve insulin sensitivity, helping to balance blood-sugar levels. Fish oils are the best source of these essential nutrients, but vegetarian options are also available – ask in the store for advice.

Specific supplement requirements

In addition to your basic plan, consider the following according to your symptoms.

For PCOS
Myo-inositol (see box, above) • n-acetylcysteine • alpha lipoic acid • chromium • magnesium
For endometriosis
Gamma linolenic acid • vitamin E • vitamin C • betacarotene • calcium D glucarate

Homocysteine

Homocysteine is an amino acid produced in your body. At high levels it can damage the lining of your arteries (the blood vessels that lead to your heart), but also other cells in your body. Studies show that elevated levels of homocysteine could be associated with poorer embryo health and an increased risk of miscarriage. A blood level that scores higher than 10 is considered to put you into the at-risk category. A high level may also predispose a woman to pre-eclampsia (dangerously high blood pressure during pregnancy that can cause complications for both the baby and the mother) and premature labour. Women with *MTHFR* gene mutations (especially the *C677T* variation),

which hamper the body's ability to break down toxins (among other functions), are much more likely to have higher-than-normal homocysteine levels. Other factors such as smoking, drug use, excess coffee and alcohol consumption, and obesity, as well as ageing, can all contribute to high homocysteine.

If a blood test reveals that you have raised levels, ask your doctor or nutritionist for advice on supplementing with vitamins B2, B6, B12 and active folic acid, as well as choline, which all work together to maintain homocysteine levels within a healthy range. Your doctor or nutritionist may advise that you take more specialist supplementations, too.

For blood-sugar balance
Alpha lipoic acid • magnesium • chromium • co-enzyme Q10 • biotin • cinnamon • protein powder

For stress
B-vitamin complex • phosphatidylserine • L-theanine • magnesium • vitamin C • adrenal supporting herbs, such as rhodiola (*Rhodiola rosea*), ashwagandha (*Withania somnifera*) or ginseng (*Panax quinquefolius*)

Many women I see in the clinic take as many as 30 supplements a day (or more!), but it's highly unlikely that anyone needs that many. However, your body is unique, so armed with the lists above, consider seeing a nutritionist who can write a programme perfectly suited to you.

Getting your body baby-ready – lifestyle

It's not just what you put into your body, but also how you live – your stress levels, activity levels, good and bad habits, the toxins in your environment and so on – that will affect your ability to have a baby.

Making lifestyle changes in order to get pregnant can be among the hardest hurdles to overcome for couples. I want to reiterate here something I said right at the start – changes need only be small to be significant. When following the guidelines, I want you to treat them with the attitude that you're being proactive but flexible. Also, please don't feel guilty if you lapse. Accept that you've had a blip and start again. If you do have a glass of wine or a cup of coffee, enjoy it!

Alcohol and your fertility

Studies show that if neither you nor your partner drinks at all you will typically get pregnant more quickly than couples who drink regularly. Alcohol can affect sperm morphology and motility, and cause free-radical damage to the DNA the sperm carries. In women, alcohol may contribute to irregular periods, irregular ovulation and luteal phase defect, reducing chances of conception.

However, I'm a realist – if alcohol forms part of your normal life, as long as you drink at the lower limits of what is recommended for your age and gender, I think you are doing okay. You are also far more likely to find lower levels sustainable than complete abstention. Try to drink fewer than six units of alcohol per week (a pint of beer is two units; a large 250ml/9fl oz glass of wine is three), and follow these guidelines:

- Both of you should try to abstain from alcohol altogether around the time of ovulation.
- Try to make sure that three or four nights a week are dry (that is, no alcohol at all).
- When you do drink alcohol, drink plenty of water, too – two glasses of water for every unit of alcohol is ideal, but try at least to match each unit with a glass of water.
- Be aware of your own character traits – if you are an all-or-nothing person, and you know you won't be able to moderate, it may in the end be better to try to cut out alcohol altogether.

Caffeine and your fertility

Some studies show links between miscarriage and caffeine consumption in women who consume five or more caffeinated drinks a day. However, researchers don't yet know for certain how caffeine levels relate to conception itself. In men, caffeine can cause sperm to become hyperactive, affecting their motility, and – for both men and women – caffeine's stimulant nature puts stress on the adrenals and causes blood sugar to start to rollercoaster with peaks and troughs.

Coffee, tea, over-the-counter medications, chocolate and fizzy drinks all contain caffeine – and don't forget that your latte or flat white might well contain more than one espresso-size shot.

The five-day fertility detox (see pages 42–4) will help you to wipe the slate clean (you may suffer caffeine-withdrawal symptoms, such as headaches, on the first few days). You may find that after the detox even the thought of caffeine seems unpalatable. But, if not, try to cut back on caffeine-containing foods and drinks during the week, treating yourself at the weekends. If you do need a shot of caffeine, take it from tea, which has much lower caffeine levels than coffee.

Smoking and fertility

Although I want to make the fertility plan manageable, smoking is a no-no. Smoking is hugely detrimental to fertility – to eggs and to sperm – not to mention the future health of the unborn child. In particular, smoking seriously depletes your body of vitamin C, which is essential to all your body's processes, and especially during pregnancy.

Your weight and your fertility

Being underweight or overweight affects fertility – and while that's especially true for women, it's true for men, too.

The most-used measure of whether or not your weight is healthy is your BMI – Body Mass Index. A female BMI of below 18.5 is underweight; 18.5–24.9 is normal; 25–29.9 is overweight; and 30 and over is obese. The ideal range for conception is 20 to 25. The ideal range for conception is 20 to 25. (There are lots of online calculators that will save you from doing the maths yourself!) While BMI is a useful guide to whether or not your weight is healthy for your size, it's worth noting that the distribution of fat in your body is also important.

Women – underweight

Being underweight is just as detrimental to fertility as being overweight. Without body fat and mass, the cascade of pituitary hormones, including FSH and LH, turns off, stopping your periods. Your body needs fat to produce oestrogen – even if you have a period, low oestrogen levels reduce your chances of ovulation. Finally, if your body perceives that you're not getting enough nutrients, it diverts its reserves to your vital organs, reducing the supply of nutrients to your organs of reproduction.

Women – overweight

Fat is virtually an organ in itself, producing hormones and chemical messengers. While you need a certain amount of it in order to produce oestrogen, too much raises oestrogen levels, causing irregular menstrual cycles, and hampers ovulation. Studies show that if an overweight woman experiencing problems conceiving can lose between 5 and 10 per cent of her weight, her fertility is likely to return.

Medicines and your fertility

First, I want to be clear that when you're trying for a baby you should not stop taking any prescribed medication unless your healthcare professional says it's okay to do so. However, it's worth knowing that some prescribed and some over-the-counter medicines may have an impact on your fertility because they can interfere with your hormone balance, in extreme cases reducing the chances of ovulation in the woman.

Medicines that you should talk to your doctor about (whether you're the man or the woman) if you want to fall pregnant, include steroids, antihistamines, antibiotics and antidepressants, as well as thyroid medication, tranquillizers, and certain blood-pressure medications. Tell your doctor you are trying for a baby and take his or her advice about how best to manage your medication in the meantime.

There is no question that many women find losing weight difficult. Undertaking the fertility detox and then following the diet plan can kick-start the process, if combined with gentle exercise three or four times a week for up to an hour each session. However, if after several months of following the programme, you see no change, I recommend seeing your medical practitioner to rule out PCOS or thyroid issues, which can make losing weight especially difficult.

Men – overweight and underweight
It may surprise you to know that fathers-to-be need to watch their weight, too. Overweight and obesity – and the associated high insulin levels – suppress the action of LH in the testes, which can significantly reduce circulating testosterone levels, affecting sperm production. Furthermore,

increased belly fat has been linked with increased aromatase. This enzyme converts testosterone to oestrogen, again affecting sperm production. In a vicious cycle, low testosterone levels result in increased abdominal fat, leading to increased aromatase activity, pushing up levels of oestrogen again and further suppressing testosterone.

Finally, an overweight man has more fat over the genital area, causing heat – which hampers the functioning of the testicles (see page 32).

Exercise and your fertility
Exercise is not just about losing weight, it is also about staying healthy. Regular exercise ensures that endorphins – feel-good hormones – circulate your body. Furthermore, it improves general circulation, including to the reproductive organs. Better circulation means that more nutrients can

Bust your stress

These are my top three tips for helping you to overcome stress. You don't need to implement all three, but if you can you will go a long way to reducing the effects of stress on your chances of conception.

- Aim for between six and eight hours of sleep a night. Too little sleep makes us irritable and exacerbates stress levels. You're far less likely to feel like getting passionate if you're overtired and grumpy. You are also more likely to crave sugar, upsetting your blood-sugar balance – which will disrupt hormone levels and result in weight gain.
- Ease your thoughts. Some form of meditation or visualization helps to break patterns of stressful thinking. One of the simplest meditations is to focus on a word or phrase that has meaning for you, such as 'calm', 'peace' or 'rest'. Practise your meditation or visualization for 20 to 30 minutes every day. Or, if meditation isn't for you, try immersing yourself in a good book, writing a journal or simply focusing fully on a certain activity (from chopping vegetables or baking bread, to mending a broken appliance or knitting). The aims are to be undisturbed and completely absorbed in your task or activity.
- Take up regular aerobic exercise. This will help burn off excess adrenaline, leaving you feeling energized, but calmer.

reach your ovaries (in a woman) or testes (in a man); and will improve your blood-sugar balance.

Try to do 30 to 60 minutes of exercise daily, but bear in mind that this needn't all be formal exercise. Take the stairs rather than the elevator to your floor at work; get off the bus two stops early and walk the rest of the way; walk to your local store and carry back your shopping rather than taking the car. These small changes, along with two or three dedicated exercise sessions each week, are far more manageable than feeling you need to get into Lycra every day.

However, your exercise timetable needs to be sustainable – please don't promise yourself that you can achieve 10 hours a week and then feel bad when you manage only four. Make your targets realistic.

Finally, many people wonder what kind of exercise they should do. Any form of exercise is worthwhile as long as it raises your heart rate. A good measure that your level is right for your state of fitness is that you should be a little out of breath, but also able to maintain a conversation while you work out. If you can't talk – slow down!

Studies show that 15 or more hours of cardiovascular exercise a week is detrimental to fertility. While this may be true, I only rarely come across this kind of problem – more typically, I see clients who exercise too little to maintain good levels of health and fertility.

Stress and your fertility

Stress depletes you of nutrients – it is one of the biggest negative factors I come across when I help couples who want to conceive. If you want to have a baby, learning techniques to help you cope with managing stress is essential.

Medical studies on levels of stress hormone and related rates of fertility are inconclusive, but I am convinced that when trying for a baby your mindset plays a huge part in creating the nurturing environment you need to conceive. It stands to reason that if your brain perceives that you are in danger – which it does when you have raised levels of adrenaline and cortisol, preparing you for fight and flight – it also perceives that now would not be a good time to bring a baby into the world.

Many people I see find that a programme of stress techniques and therapies – including hypnotherapy, acupuncture, massage and meditation – can be very effective at dealing with stress. However, relieving stress does not necessarily require formal techniques. Take a look at the box (opposite), for my top tips on stress-relief.

Dealing with the unpredictable

Modern life tends to be increasingly stressful, but when it doesn't happen straightaway the most primal human act of getting pregnant can be stressful, too. There is very little that is predictable about getting pregnant. It could happen this month, next month, next year, or even beyond, and it is so important that couples remember to stay positive.

In the clinic I urge couples to remember how much their baby is, first and foremost, an expression of their commitment to each other, not the reason for their commitment to each other. Try to make sure that you both get enough sleep – being tired is the enemy of feeling relaxed and calm, and sexy. Take time out together every week, away from the bedroom and the need for babymaking. A long walk at the weekend, playing a sport together and trips to the movies or a concert are all ways to remember that you came together for a reason that had nothing to do with having a baby. Feeling relaxed in yourselves and with each other is an important part of the process and will keep the passion alight.

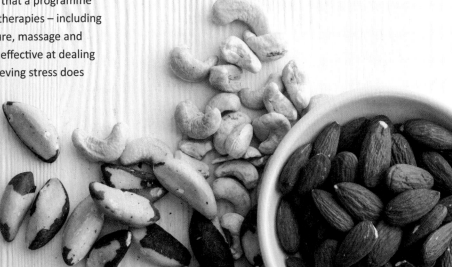

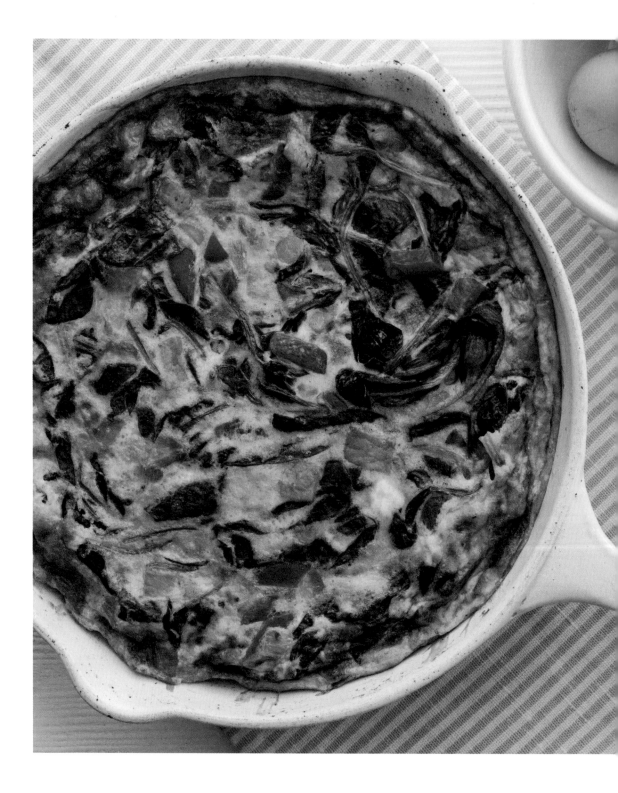

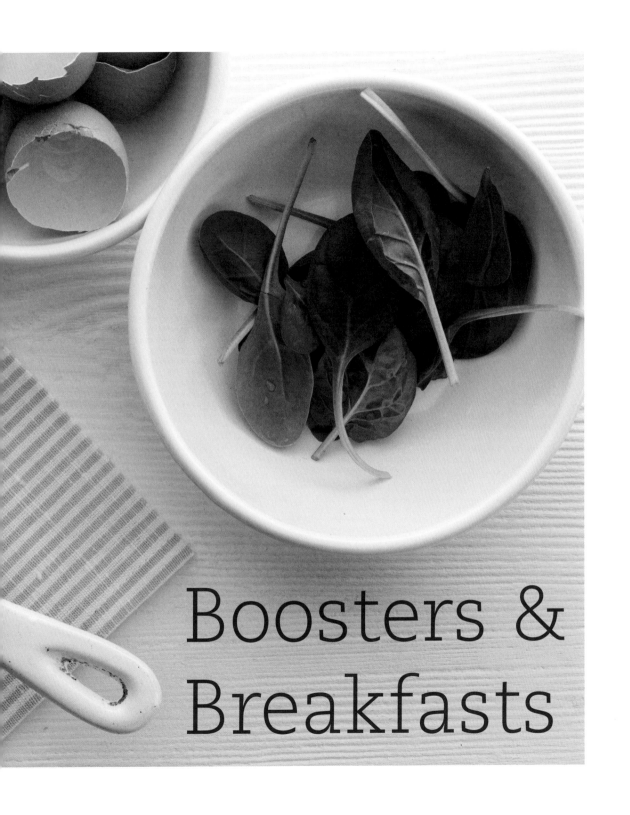

Boosters & Breakfasts

The Deep Green Cleanse

Rich in alkalizing greens and incredibly hydrating, this juice is great for cleansing the body and replenishing minerals often low in our diets, particularly magnesium.

2 large handfuls of spinach
  leaves or kale

1 cucumber

1 lemon, peeled

3 celery stalks

2 apples

ice, to serve (optional)

1 Put all the ingredients through an electric juicer. Serve immediately with ice, if using.

SERVES: 2 • PREPARATION TIME: 5 MINUTES
NUTRITIONAL INFORMATION PER SERVING: PROTEIN 0.9G CARBOHYDRATE 10.1G, OF WHICH SUGARS 9.9G FAT 0.5G, OF WHICH SATURATES 0.1G KCALS 51

Green Energizer

1 large handful of spinach leaves

1 banana, chopped and frozen

150g/5½oz/scant 1 cup peeled,
  cored and chopped pineapple

1 tsp ground flaxseed

1 tsp honey

1 tsp super-green powder, such as
  chlorella or spirulina (optional)

½ cucumber, chopped

400ml/14fl oz/generous 1½ cups
  coconut water or cold green tea

1 Put all the ingredients in a blender or food processor and process until thick and creamy. Serve immediately.

SERVES: 2 • PREPARATION TIME: 5 MINUTES
NUTRITIONAL INFORMATION PER SERVING: PROTEIN 4.4G CARBOHYDRATE 29.7G, OF WHICH SUGARS 21G FAT 2.1G, OF WHICH SATURATES 0.2G KCALS 154

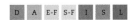

Avocado Antioxidant Fruit Blend

Packed with healthy fats and plenty of vitamins, this delicious creamy shake will help protect the body from oxidative damage.

1 mango, peeled, pitted and chopped

1 handful of strawberries

1 ripe avocado, peeled, pitted and chopped

1 tsp acai berry powder (optional)

250ml/9fl oz/1 cup pomegranate juice

150ml/5fl oz/scant ⅔ cup water or coconut water

1 Put all the ingredients in a blender or food processor and process until smooth. Add a little water if needed to thin. Serve immediately.

SERVES: 2 • PREPARATION TIME: 5 MINUTES
NUTRITIONAL INFORMATION PER SERVING: PROTEIN 2G CARBOHYDRATE 26.4G, OF WHICH SUGARS 25.6G FAT 10.7G, OF WHICH SATURATES 2.1G KCALS 210

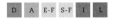

B Booster

1 large raw beetroot

2 carrots

2 apples

2 oranges, peeled

a small piece of root ginger (optional)

1 Put all the ingredients through an electric juicer and serve immediately.

SERVES: 2 • PREPARATION TIME: 5 MINUTES
NUTRITIONAL INFORMATION PER SERVING: PROTEIN 2.3G CARBOHYDRATE 24.4G, OF WHICH SUGARS 23.4G FAT 0.4G, OF WHICH SATURATES 0.1G KCALS 104

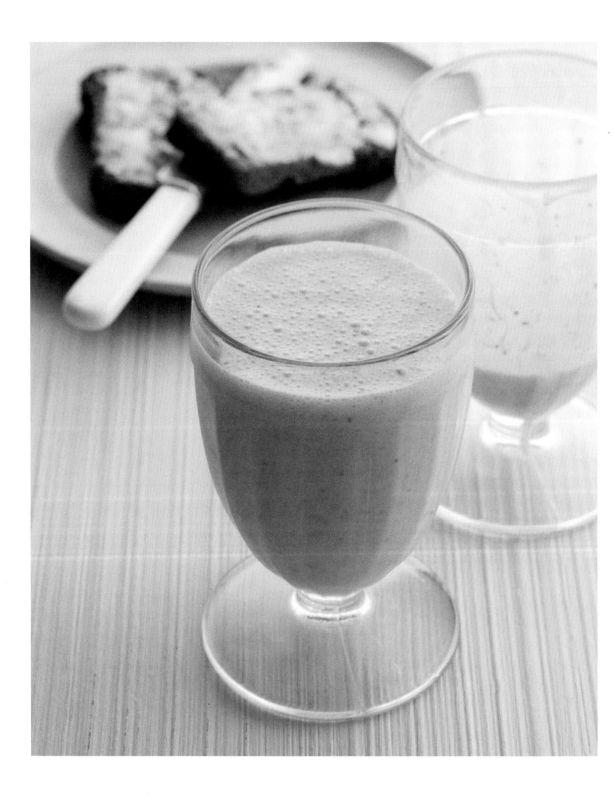

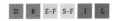

Strawberry Kefir

This fruity shake is made with kefir, an ancient cultured food that is packed with an array of beneficial bacteria useful for improving digestive health. The addition of strawberries also provides plenty of vitamins and nutrients to help protect the body from damage.

400ml/14fl oz/generous 1½ cups milk kefir

1 large banana, chopped

225g/8oz/1½ cups strawberries, hulled and frozen

1 tsp vanilla extract

1–2 tbsp honey

1 Put all the ingredients in a blender or food processor and process until smooth. Serve immediately.

SERVES: 2 • PREPARATION TIME: 5 MINUTES
NUTRITIONAL INFORMATION PER SERVING: PROTEIN 10.4G CARBOHYDRATE 32.7G, OF WHICH SUGARS 23.1G FAT 1.8, OF WHICH SATURATES 0.1G KCALS 195

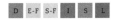

Stress-Busting Mocha

75g/2½oz/scant ½ cup cashew nuts

250ml/9fl oz/1 cup coconut water

1 tsp maca powder

1 banana, chopped and frozen

2 tbsp raw cacao powder

1 tbsp chia seeds

1 tbsp coconut sugar or honey

1 tsp vanilla extract

2 large handfuls of crushed ice

1 Put the cashews and coconut water in a blender or food processor and process until smooth. Add the remaining ingredients, except the ice, and process until smooth. Blend in the ice and serve immediately.

SERVES: 2 • PREPARATION TIME: 5 MINUTES
NUTRITIONAL INFORMATION PER SERVING: PROTEIN 12.2G CARBOHYDRATE 42.5G, OF WHICH SUGARS 18.3G FAT 22G, OF WHICH SATURATES 4.6G KCALS 416

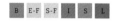

Fruit & Mango Cream Parfait

This delicious sweet parfait combines antioxidant-packed berries and rich mango cream to provide plenty of protein to help stabilize blood sugars throughout the morning. For a change, a medley of citrus fruits could be used instead of the berries. The mango cream can be prepared in advance and kept in the fridge for 2–3 days and is delicious served with poached fruit. If you have time, soak the seeds and nuts first, which softens them and can help improve digestibility.

1 tbsp unsweetened coconut flakes

1 tbsp sunflower seeds

1 tbsp pumpkin seeds

a pinch of ground cinnamon

a pinch of sea salt

150g/5½oz/heaped 1 cup mixed berries (such as blueberries, cherries or raspberries)

MANGO VANILLA CREAM

60g/2¼oz/heaped ⅓ cup almonds

1 small mango, peeled, pitted and diced

3 tbsp lucuma powder (optional)

1 tsp vanilla extract

1 In a bowl, mix together the coconut flakes, sunflower seeds, pumpkin seeds, cinnamon and salt.

2 Put all the ingredients for the mango vanilla cream in a blender or food processor with 100ml/3½fl oz/generous ⅓ cup water and process until smooth.

3 Spoon a quarter of the mango cream into each of two glasses. Top with a spoonful of mixed berries and sprinkle over a little of the coconut seed mixture. Repeat the layer, finishing with a sprinkling of the coconut and seeds.

SERVES: 2 • PREPARATION TIME: 10 MINUTES

NUTRITIONAL INFORMATION PER SERVING: PROTEIN 12.1G CARBOHYDRATE 37G, OF WHICH SUGARS 17.8G
FAT 26G, OF WHICH SATURATES 16.3G KCALS 436

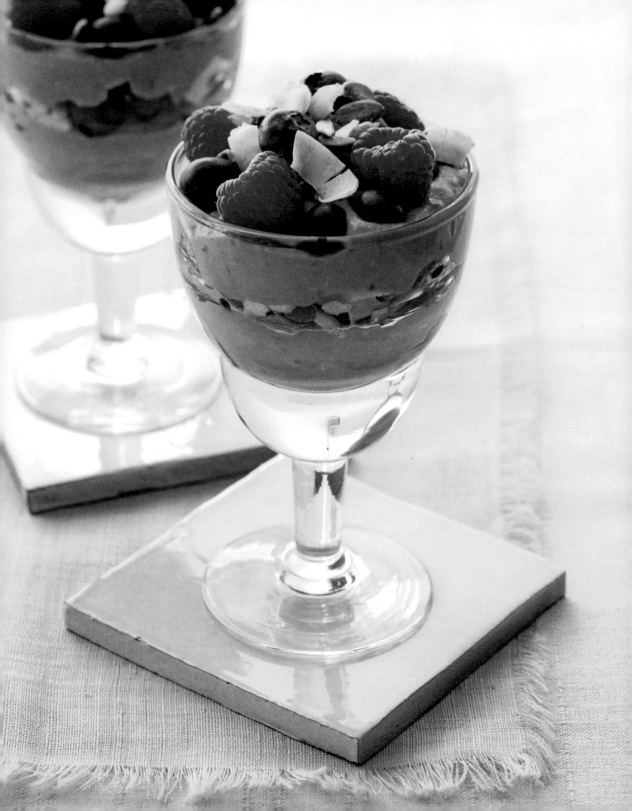

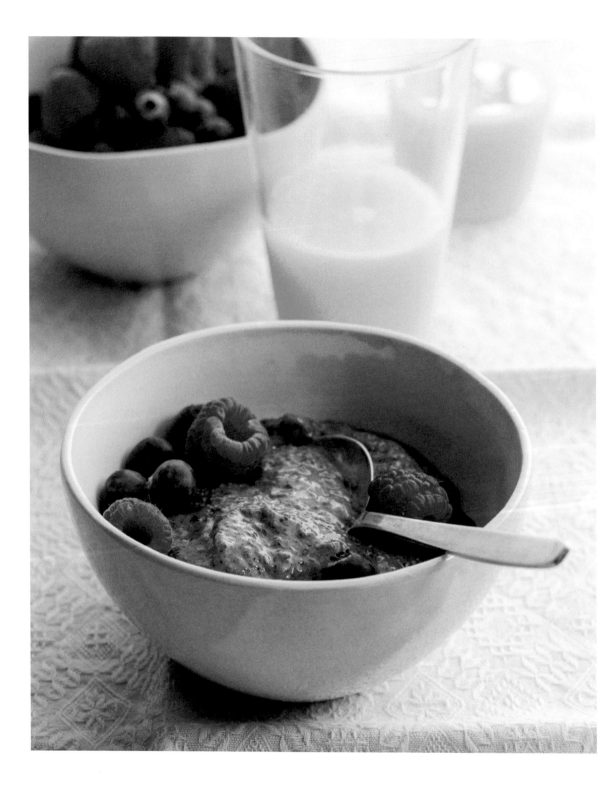

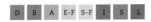

Super Berry Chia Pudding

Prepare this delicious, antioxidant-packed dish the night before to allow the chia seeds to swell and thicken the pudding. Chia seeds are a real superfood: packed with protein, omega-3 fats and soluble fibre, they provide plenty of slow-releasing energy to keep you fuelled all morning and help to avoid energy dips and cravings.

1 banana, chopped

125g/4½oz/heaped ¾ cup blueberries, plus extra to serve

200g/7oz/scant 1⅓ cups raspberries, plus extra to serve

250ml/9fl oz/1 cup semi-skimmed milk or milk alternative (such as coconut milk or almond milk)

6 tbsp chia seeds

2 tsp honey

2 tsp acai berry powder (optional)

1 Put all the ingredients in a blender or food processor and process until incorporated. Put the pudding in the fridge and let it soak overnight.

2 In the morning, serve the pudding topped with berries.

SERVES: 2 • PREPARATION TIME: 5 MINUTES, PLUS OVERNIGHT SOAKING

NUTRITIONAL INFORMATION PER SERVING: PROTEIN 11.3 CARBOHYDRATE 41.8G, OF WHICH SUGARS 27.9G
FAT 12.7G, OF WHICH SATURATES 2.4G KCALS 319

Quick Grain-Free Almond Bread

This is a grain-free, protein-packed speedy bread. Sweet and creamy, it is delicious served warm from the oven, but will keep in the fridge for a couple of days or can be frozen, too. Add a handful of raisins to make it a wonderfully moist tea loaf. Almonds provide plenty of protein and soluble fibre and are also rich in vitamin E – a powerful antioxidant that has been shown to increase fertility in both men and women. It's always a good idea to eat a handful of raw almonds every day as a snack while trying to conceive.

olive oil or coconut oil,
  for greasing

1 apple, peeled, cored and
  chopped

2 tbsp apple juice

125g/4½oz/½ cup almond
  nut butter

4 tbsp honey

2 eggs

1 tbsp vanilla extract

2 tbsp ground cinnamon

½ tsp sea salt

1 Preheat the oven to 180°C/350°F/Gas 4 and grease a 20cm/8in square baking tin or 450g/1lb loaf tin with oil.
2 In a food processor, combine the apple, apple juice and almond butter and pulse until well blended. Add the honey, eggs, vanilla extract, cinnamon and salt and pulse to combine.
3 Pour the batter into the prepared tin and bake for 35 minutes until golden and firm to the touch.

MAKES: 1 LOAF (6 SLICES) • PREPARATION TIME: 10 MINUTES • COOKING TIME: 35 MINUTES
NUTRITIONAL INFORMATION PER SLICE: PROTEIN 5.2G CARBOHYDRATE 11.7G, OF WHICH SUGARS 11G
FAT 9.5G, OF WHICH SATURATES 2.4G KCALS 154

Overnight Muesli

A delicious soaked muesli which can be prepared the night before to make a simple no-fuss breakfast option when time is short. Coconut is rich in an array of vitamins and minerals, and can also help support the immune system. Serve topped with fresh berries.

2 tbsp raw cacao nibs

2 tbsp unsweetened dried berries, goji berries or raisins

2 tbsp sunflower seeds

2 tbsp unsweetened coconut flakes

60g/2¼oz/⅔ cup rolled oats

150ml/5fl oz/scant ⅔ cup full-fat milk or milk alternative, plus extra to taste

1 apple, cored and diced

berries, to serve (optional)

1 Put all the ingredients in a small container and stir to mix. Put the muesli in the fridge and let it soak overnight.

2 In the morning, stir again and add more milk, if you like. Serve cold topped with berries, if using.

SERVES: 2 • PREPARATION TIME: 5 MINUTES, PLUS OVERNIGHT SOAKING
NUTRITIONAL INFORMATION PER SERVING: PROTEIN 12G CARBOHYDRATE 46.9G, OF WHICH SUGARS 20G
FAT 29.2G, OF WHICH SATURATES 15G KCALS 482

Protein Boost Seeded Granola

This is a healthy version of the classic breakfast option, with an array of seeds to provide plenty of healthy fats. Research has found that Brazil nuts can assist male fertility as well as boost testosterone. You can vary the ingredients according to what you have available. This will keep in an airtight container for 1–2 weeks.

115g/4oz/¾ cup Brazil nuts

115g/4oz/¾ cup almonds

115g/4oz/2 cups unsweetened coconut flakes

60g/2¼oz/½ cup raw cacao nibs

60g/2¼oz/½ cup pumpkin seeds

60g/2¼oz/½ cup sunflower seeds

60g/2¼oz/⅔ cup shelled hemp seeds

1 apple, cored and chopped

75g/2½oz/heaped ⅓ cup soft pitted dates

2 tbsp honey or maple syrup

2 tbsp coconut oil or olive oil

1 scoop of vanilla protein powder (optional)

2 tbsp lucuma powder (optional)

1 tsp vanilla extract

1 tsp ground cinnamon

½ tsp sea salt

60g/2¼oz/⅔ cup goji berries or unsweetened dried cherries

milk or milk alternative, or yogurt, to serve

1 Preheat the oven to 160°C/315°F/Gas 2–3 and line a baking sheet with baking parchment.

2 Put the nuts, coconut flakes, cacao nibs and seeds in a food processor and process to coarsely chop. Transfer them to a large mixing bowl.

3 Put the apple, dates, honey, coconut oil, protein powder, if using, lucuma powder, if using, vanilla extract, cinnamon and salt in a food processor and process to form a thick paste. Pour the paste over the nuts and seeds and stir to combine well.

4 Spread the mixture onto the prepared baking sheet and bake for 20 minutes. Turn down the oven to 110°C/225°F/Gas ½ and bake for a further 30 minutes, or until the mixture is dry and golden. Leave to cool, then stir in the berries. Store in an airtight container. Serve with a splash of milk or yogurt.

Makes: 8 servings • **Preparation time:** 10 minutes • **Cooking time:** 50 minutes
Nutritional information per serving: Protein 10.6g **Carbohydrate** 19.4g, of which sugars 13g
Fat 29g, of which saturates 10.6g **Kcals** 376

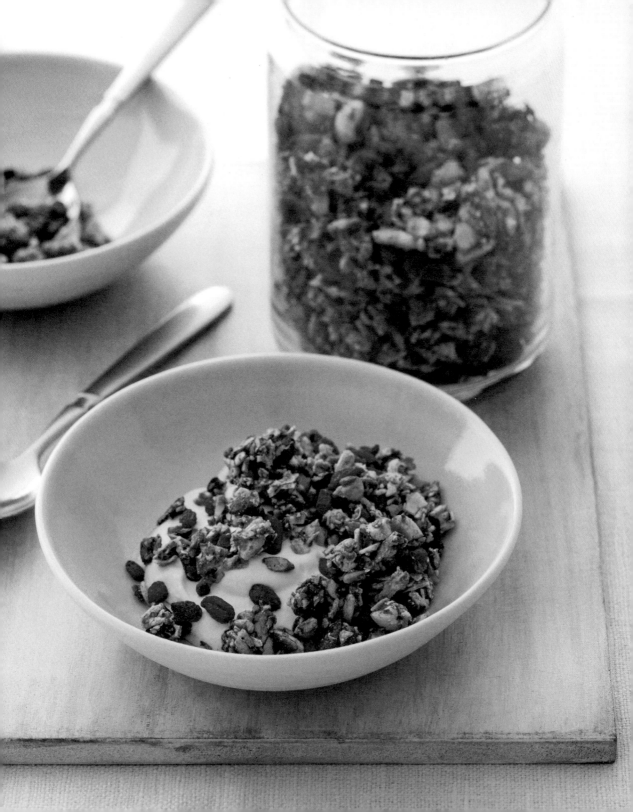

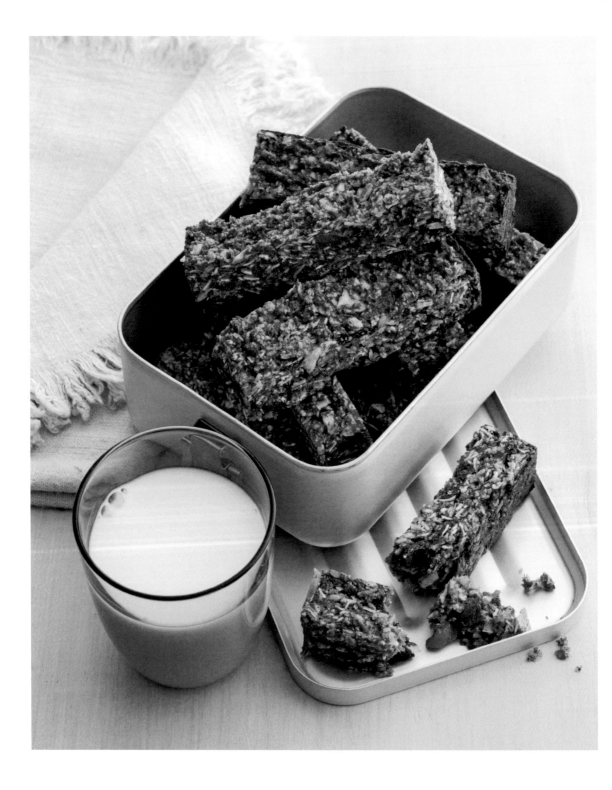

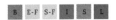

Breakfast Wake-Up Bars

A healthy cereal bar is perfect if you don't have time for a sit-down breakfast. These bars contain plenty of protein with the addition of nuts and seeds to keep blood-sugar levels stable throughout the morning. The addition of maca powder is a great way to support the adrenal glands if you're feeling stressed. Oats are high in slow-releasing carbohydrate and rich in soluble fibre to keep you feeling fuller for longer and avoid mid-morning energy dips. They also contain plenty of vitamin E and energizing B-vitamins, as well as beta glucans that support immune health.

olive oil or coconut oil, for greasing

125g/4½oz/heaped ¾ cup cashew nuts

150g/5½oz/1½ cups rolled oats

60g/2¼oz/heaped 1 cup unsweetened coconut flakes

1 tbsp maca powder (optional)

1 tbsp shelled hemp seeds

1 tbsp sunflower seeds

1 tbsp flaxseeds

60g/2¼oz/¼ cup chopped ready-to-eat dried apricots

60g/2¼oz/⅔ cup goji berries

a pinch of sea salt

60g/2¼oz/¼ cup almond or cashew nut butter

60g/2¼oz/scant ¼ cup honey

200g/7oz/heaped 1 cup soft pitted dates, chopped

1 teaspoon vanilla extract

1 Preheat the oven to 180°C/350°F/Gas 4 and grease a shallow 20cm/8in square baking tin with oil.

2 Put the cashews in a food processor and process until fine. Add the oats and coconut flakes and pulse to break up slightly. Transfer to a mixing bowl and stir in the maca powder, if using, seeds, apricots, goji berries and salt.

3 In a food processor, blend together the nut butter, honey, dates and vanilla extract to form a paste. Mix the paste into the dry ingredients. Spread the mixture into the prepared baking tin. Bake for 20–25 minutes, or until slightly golden. Leave to cool in the tin, then cut into 16 bars.

MAKES: 16 BARS • PREPARATION TIME: 15 MINUTES • COOKING TIME: 25 MINUTES
NUTRITIONAL INFORMATION PER BAR: PROTEIN 4.9G CARBOHYDRATE 23.4G, OF WHICH SUGARS 15.8G
FAT 10.3G, OF WHICH SATURATES 3.4G KCALS 206

E-F S-F

Lemon Blueberry Muesli Muffins

These sensational low-sugar muffins, full of nuts and seeds, are perfect as a healthy option for breakfast, but equally delicious as a healthy snack. They are made with xylitol – a sweetener that raises blood sugar levels less than regular sugar – and wholemeal flour, which is a slow-releasing carbohydrate that helps to balance blood sugar. Whole grains are also rich in soluble fibre and contain plenty of B-vitamins, which are important for producing healthy eggs and sperm. Using frozen blueberries creates a colder batter but fresh blueberries can also be used.

4 tbsp olive oil, plus extra for greasing

150g/5½oz/1 cup wholemeal self-raising flour

2 tsp baking powder

a pinch of sea salt

1 tsp ground cinnamon

115g/4oz/scant 1 cup low-sugar muesli

1 tbsp ground flaxseed

75g/2½oz/heaped ⅓ cup xylitol

3 eggs

zest of 1 lemon

1 tbsp lemon juice

125ml/4fl oz/½ cup semi-skimmed milk or milk alternative

115g/4oz/¾ cup frozen blueberries

1 Preheat the oven to 180°C/350°F/Gas 4 and line eight holes of a muffin tin with paper cases.

2 Put the flour, baking powder, salt, cinnamon and muesli in a large mixing bowl.

3 Put the remaining ingredients, except the blueberries, into a food processor or blender and process until smooth. Pour into the flour mixture and beat well to form a thick batter, then gently stir in the blueberries.

4 Spoon the mixture evenly into the paper cases and bake for 15–20 minutes until golden brown and firm on top. Leave to cool in the tins for 5 minutes before turning out onto a wire rack to cool completely.

MAKES: 8 muffins • PREPARATION TIME: 10 MINUTES • COOKING TIME: 20 MINUTES
NUTRITIONAL INFORMATION PER MUFFIN: PROTEIN 7.2G CARBOHYDRATE 31.7G, OF WHICH SUGARS 13.2G
FAT 9.2G, OF WHICH SATURATES 8G KCALS 225

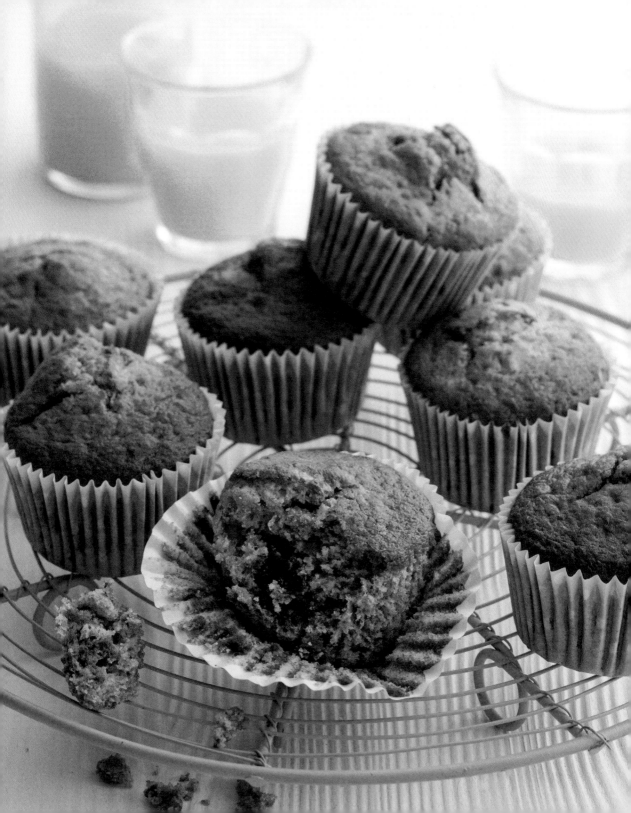

Bacon & Spinach Frittata

Instead of a greasy fry-up, try this fabulous frittata. Perfect for a weekend brunch, this dish packs in plenty of energizing iron and magnesium-rich spinach, too. Studies have shown that starting the day with a high-fat, high-protein breakfast such as bacon and eggs improves the metabolism and prevents blood-sugar dips that can lead to snacking. Bacon also provides plenty of B-vitamins for energy production, and selenium which is important for sperm health and fertility.

8 eggs

1 tbsp coconut oil or olive oil

1 small onion, diced

4 bacon rashers, chopped

½ red pepper, deseeded and chopped

100g/3½oz baby spinach leaves

sea salt and ground black pepper

1 Preheat the grill to high. Whisk the eggs in a bowl and season with salt and pepper.

2 Heat half of the oil in a flameproof frying pan. Add the onion, bacon and red pepper and sauté for 2–3 minutes until the bacon is beginning to crisp. Stir in the spinach and allow to wilt, then add the vegetables and bacon to the eggs.

3 Add the remaining oil to the pan and pour in the egg mixture. Cook over a low heat for 2–3 minutes until the bottom of the frittata is beginning to set. Put the pan under the grill and cook for 5–6 minutes until golden on top, then serve.

Pictured on page 56

SERVES: 4 • PREPARATION TIME: 10 MINUTES • COOKING TIME: 14 MINUTES

NUTRITIONAL INFORMATION PER SERVING: PROTEIN 15.8G CARBOHYDRATE 2.1G, OF WHICH SUGARS 1.7G

FAT 17.3G, OF WHICH SATURATES 4.7G KCALS 227

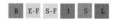

Poached Eggs with Asparagus & Toasted Seeds

This is a delicious and healthy cooked-breakfast option. Protein rich and nourishing, it is packed with healthy fats and nutrients to support fertility. Free-range and organic eggs contain a higher omega 3 content and the addition of seeds provides additional omega-3 and omega-6 fats. Asparagus is considered an aphrodisiac; it is rich in folic acid, a B-vitamin that helps with the production of healthy sperm in men and in the prevention of neural tube defects, such as spina bifida, in the foetus.

2 tbsp pumpkin seeds
2 tbsp sunflower seeds
2 tbsp sesame seeds
2 tsp soy sauce
8 asparagus spears
1 tbsp white wine vinegar
2 eggs

1 Heat a dry frying pan over a medium heat and add the seeds. Toast for 1–2 minutes, then add the soy sauce. Stir until the seeds have soaked up the liquid and turned lightly golden. Remove from the heat and leave to cool.

2 Bring a saucepan of water to the boil, add the asparagus spears and cook for 1–2 minutes, then drain.

3 For the poached eggs, bring a small pan of water to a gentle simmer and add the vinegar. Stir the simmering water, then carefully crack the eggs into the water. Poach for 2–3 minutes, or until the eggs are cooked to your liking, then carefully remove from the pan using a slotted spoon and drain on kitchen paper.

4 To serve, divide the asparagus spears between two plates. Place a poached egg on top of each and sprinkle over the toasted seeds.

SERVES: 2 • PREPARATION TIME: 5 MINUTES • COOKING TIME: 8 MINUTES
NUTRITIONAL INFORMATION PER SERVING: PROTEIN 16.3G CARBOHYDRATE 5.6G, OF WHICH SUGARS 1.2G
FAT 28.2G, OF WHICH SATURATES 5.2G KCALS 343

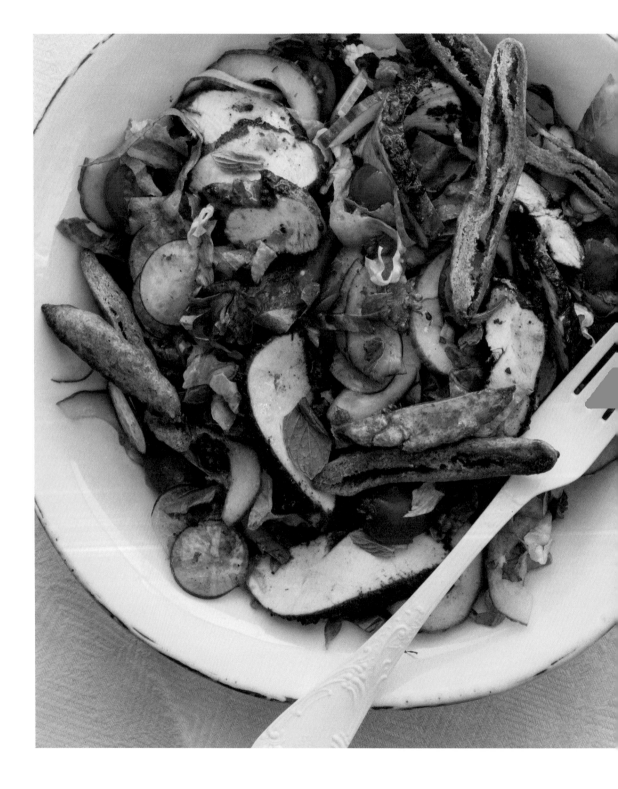

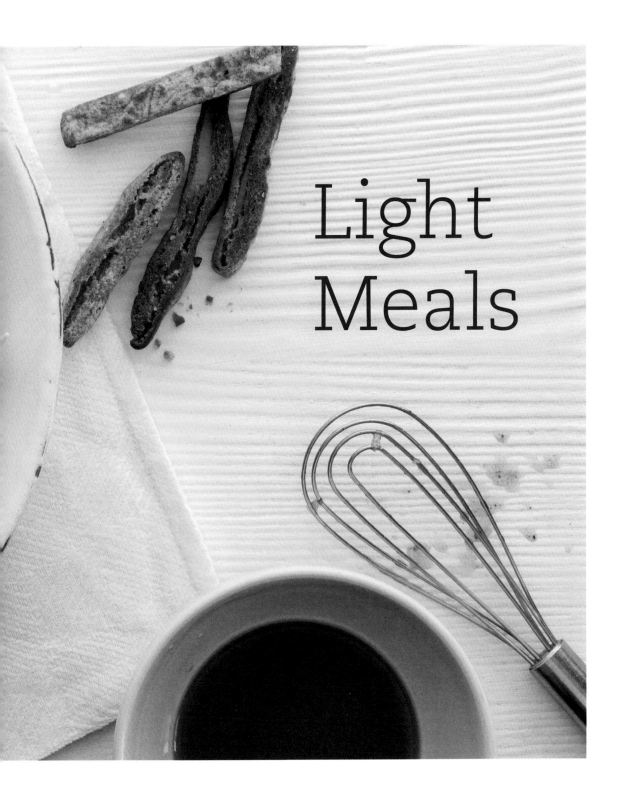

Light
Meals

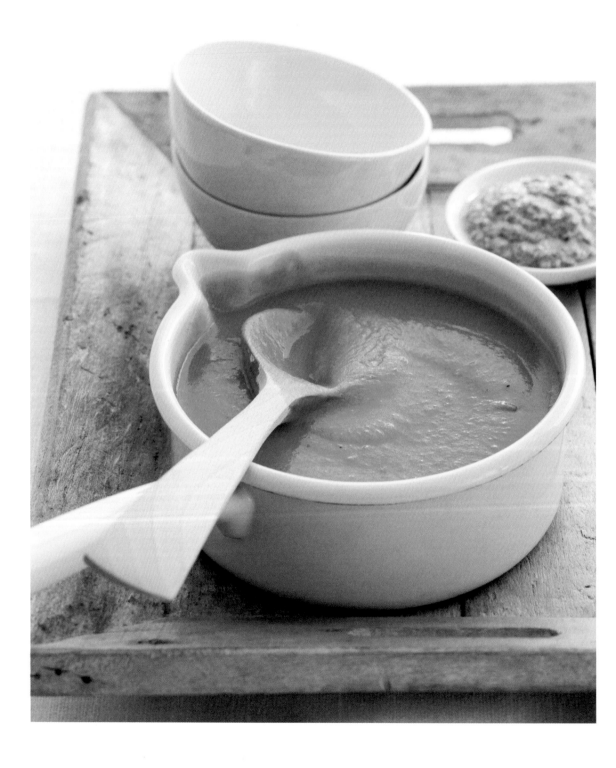

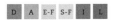

Roasted Butternut Squash & Ginger Soup with Hemp Pesto

1 red onion, cut into wedges

3 garlic cloves, peeled

1cm/½in piece of root ginger, peeled

1 butternut squash, about 750g/1lb 10oz, peeled, deseeded and cut into 2.5cm/1in cubes

1 sweet potato, peeled and cut into chunks

60ml/2fl oz/¼ cup olive oil

1 tsp ground cinnamon

700ml/24fl oz/scant 3 cups hot vegetable stock

HEMP PESTO

60g/2¼oz/⅔ cup shelled hemp seeds

2 garlic cloves, crushed

½ tsp sea salt

1 large handful of basil leaves

3 tbsp nutritional yeast flakes

2 tbsp lemon juice

2 tbsp extra virgin olive oil

2 tbsp hemp seed oil

ground black pepper

Roasting the vegetables adds a wonderful sweet, caramelized flavour to this soup, and makes it incredibly simple to prepare. Packed full of betacarotene, garlic and ginger, this is a fabulous anti-inflammatory, immune-supporting dish. Adding the hemp pesto provides omega-3 essential fats, while butternut squash is an excellent source of antioxidants and vitamin A, which is particularly important for female reproductive health.

1 To make the hemp pesto, put the hemp seeds in a food processor and process until fine. Add the remaining ingredients and process again to form a thick paste. Store in the fridge until required.

2 Preheat the oven to 200°C/400°F/Gas 6. Put the onion, garlic cloves, ginger, butternut squash and sweet potato in a roasting tin. Drizzle with the olive oil and sprinkle with the cinnamon. Roast for 40 minutes, or until tender.

3 Put the roasted vegetables and vegetable stock in a blender or food processor and process until smooth – you may have to do this in two batches. Transfer to a saucepan and season to taste with salt and pepper. Warm in the pan for a couple of minutes, then ladle into bowls and serve with a dollop of hemp pesto.

SERVES: 4 • PREPARATION TIME: 10 MINUTES • COOKING TIME: 45 MINUTES
NUTRITIONAL INFORMATION PER SERVING: PROTEIN 10.1G CARBOHYDRATE 25.2G, OF WHICH SUGARS 10.7G
FAT 33.2G, OF WHICH SATURATES 3.9G KCALS 440

Chunky Minestrone Soup

This hearty, chunky soup is packed with an array of nutrient-rich vegetables – perfect for when you crave comforting, warming foods. Vary the vegetables according to the season – in the spring try adding asparagus, broad beans or courgettes. For additional protein try adding a little ham or cooked bacon.

2 tbsp olive oil, plus extra to serve

1 red onion, chopped

2 carrots, peeled and roughly chopped

3 celery sticks, chopped

2 garlic cloves, crushed

2 leeks, sliced

1 small potato, peeled and diced

400g/14oz/scant 1⅔ cups tinned chopped tomatoes

600ml/21fl oz/scant 2½ cups chicken or vegetable stock

½ Savoy cabbage, shredded, or a bunch of Swiss chard, stems removed and leaves chopped

410g/14½oz tinned cannellini beans, drained and rinsed

2 tbsp chopped parsley leaves

sea salt and ground black pepper

2 tbsp grated Parmesan, to serve (optional)

1 Heat the olive oil in a large saucepan over a low heat and sauté the onion, carrots, celery, garlic, leeks and potato for about 10 minutes. Add the tomatoes and stock and simmer for 10 minutes. Add the cabbage and beans and cook for a further 10 minutes, then season to taste with salt and pepper.

2 Stir in the parsley and serve the soup hot, sprinkled with Parmesan, if you like, and a drizzle of olive oil.

Serves: 4 • Preparation time: 10 minutes • Cooking time: 30 minutes
Nutritional information per serving: Protein 9.3g Carbohydrate 17.4g, of which sugars 7.7g
Fat 7.9g, of which saturates 2.2g Kcals 178

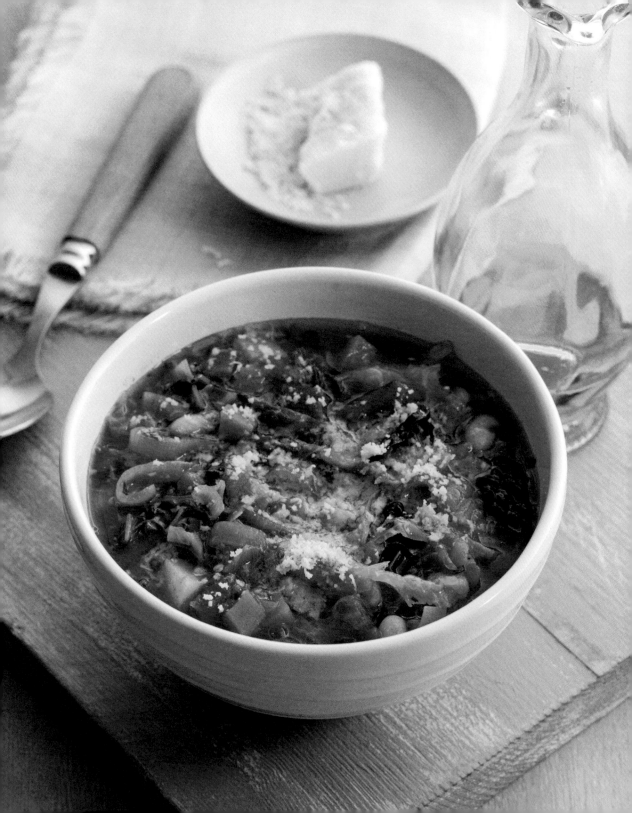

Broccoli, Fennel & Pear Soup

This is a beautiful, light yet creamy-tasting soup – perfect for detox days. The addition of pear provides a natural sweetness and is rich in pectin to help remove toxins from the body. Fennel provides good support to the liver for cleansing, while broccoli, fennel and pear are all good sources of potassium, to help alkalize the body.

1 tbsp olive oil, plus extra to serve

1 small onion, chopped

1 garlic clove, finely chopped

150g/5½oz broccoli, chopped

1 fennel bulb, trimmed and chopped

600ml/21fl oz/scant 2½ cups vegetable stock

1 pear, cored and chopped

sea salt and ground black pepper

1 Heat the oil in a large saucepan over a medium heat and sauté the onion and garlic for 2–3 minutes.

2 Add the broccoli and fennel to the pan and stir to coat in the oil. Add the vegetable stock and bring to the boil, then turn the heat down and leave to simmer for 20–25 minutes until the vegetables are tender. Transfer the soup to a blender or food processor, add the pear and process until smooth and creamy.

3 Transfer to a saucepan and season to taste with salt and pepper. Warm in the pan for a couple of minutes, then ladle into bowls and serve with a drizzle of olive oil.

SERVES: 2 • PREPARATION TIME: 10 MINUTES • COOKING TIME: 30 MINUTES
NUTRITIONAL INFORMATION PER SERVING: PROTEIN 4.5G CARBOHYDRATE 9.7G, OF WHICH SUGARS 9.3G
FAT 5.8G, OF WHICH SATURATES 0.8G KCALS 110

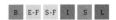

Lebanese Fattoush Salad with Sumac-Roasted Chicken

2 skinless chicken breasts

2 tbsp olive oil, plus extra to cook the pittas

juice of ½ lemon

1 tbsp sumac

1 wholemeal pitta bread

1 Romaine lettuce, shredded

200g/7oz/1⅓ cups cherry tomatoes, halved

1 cucumber, halved lengthways, deseeded and sliced

8 radishes, thinly sliced

½ red pepper, deseeded and cut into chunks

1 handful of parsley leaves, chopped

1 handful of mint leaves, chopped

sea salt and ground black pepper

LEMON & SUMAC DRESSING

juice and zest of 1 lemon

4 tbsp olive oil

1 tbsp flaxseed oil or omega-blend oil

1 tbsp honey

½ tsp sumac

Pictured on page 76

This Middle Eastern-style salad is tossed with an omega-rich dressing and contains an array of vegetables and crispy pieces of wholemeal pitta. It is also protein-packed and full of flavour. Sumac is a ground spice made from dried berries – you should be able to find it in Middle Eastern stores. If you can't, you can add 1 tablespoon grated lemon zest instead. Chicken is a great source of B-vitamins to help combat the effects of stress by keeping your brain running smoothly and your energy high.

1 Put the chicken in a shallow non-reactive dish. Mix together the 2 tablespoons olive oil, lemon juice and sumac and pour over the chicken. Cover and leave to marinate in the fridge for 30 minutes.

2 To make the pitta pieces, preheat the oven to 200°C/400°F/Gas 6. Cut the pittas into 1cm/½in wide strips, toss them with a little olive oil and season with salt and pepper. Lay them on a baking tray and bake for 5–7 minutes until golden, then leave to cool.

3 Turn up the oven to 220°C/425°F/Gas 7. Put the chicken in a roasting tin and cook for 13–15 minutes until cooked through and the juices run clear. Leave to cool, then slice.

4 Mix all the dressing ingredients together in a small bowl and season to taste.

5 Combine the lettuce, tomatoes, cucumber, radishes, red pepper and herbs in a large bowl and toss together. Top with the chicken and pitta pieces and drizzle over the dressing to serve.

SERVES: 4 • PREPARATION TIME: 15 MINUTES, PLUS 30 MINUTES MARINATING • COOKING TIME: 22 MINUTES

NUTRITIONAL INFORMATION PER SERVING: PROTEIN 23G CARBOHYDRATE 16.6G, OF WHICH SUGARS 7.6G

FAT 22.1G, OF WHICH SATURATES 3.2G KCALS 359

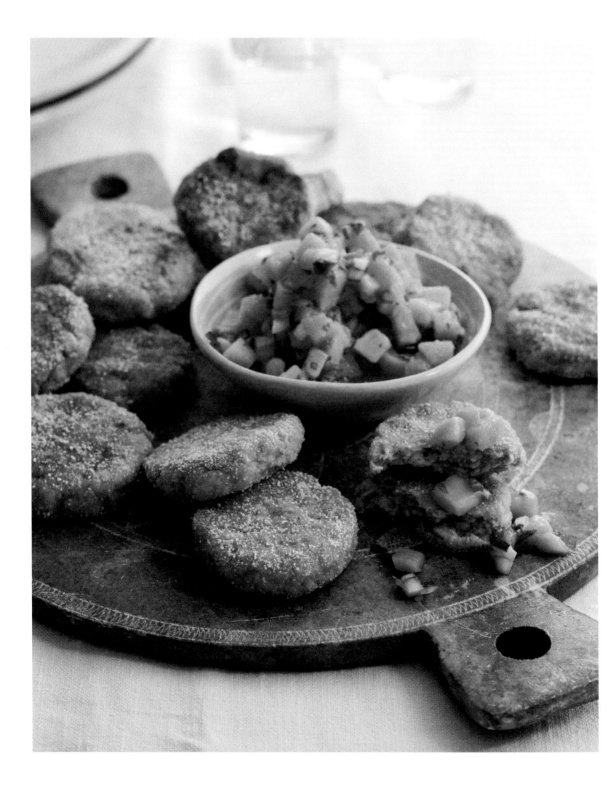

Spiced Chicken Patties with Mango & Coriander Salsa

2 boneless, skinless chicken breasts, chopped

2 tbsp fish sauce

1 tbsp soy sauce

1 tsp peeled and grated root ginger

1 garlic clove, crushed

a pinch of sea salt

a pinch of smoked paprika

100g/3½oz/⅔ cup polenta

olive oil or coconut oil, for frying

leafy green salad, to serve

MANGO & CORIANDER SALSA

1 small red chilli, deseeded and finely diced

½ red onion, finely diced

1 small ripe mango, peeled, pitted and finely diced

juice of 2 limes

1 handful of coriander leaves, chopped

sea salt and ground black pepper

These light chicken patties are spiked with ginger and garlic and accompanied by a sweet, tangy salsa. Coating the cakes in polenta gives them a delicious crispy crumb. They can be served cold and make an easy packed-lunch option. For additional healthy fats, add some diced avocado to the salsa. Coriander is exceptionally rich in phytonutrients and is often used to help support cleansing and liver detoxification. Rich in volatile oil, it is known to possess anti-microbial properties, protecting the body from infections.

1 To make the mango and coriander salsa, combine all the ingredients in a non-reactive bowl.

2 Put the chicken breasts in a food processor and pulse to break up slightly. Add all the remaining ingredients except the polenta and process to combine.

3 Sprinkle the polenta on a plate. Scoop out walnut-sized pieces of the chicken mixture and shape into small, round cakes. Press the cakes into the polenta all over to coat.

4 Heat the oil in a large frying pan over a medium heat. Brown the patties for about 2–3 minutes on each side until cooked through, then drain on kitchen paper. Serve with the salsa and a leafy green salad.

SERVES: 4 • PREPARATION TIME: 15 MINUTES • COOKING TIME: 6 MINUTES

NUTRITIONAL INFORMATION PER SERVING: PROTEIN 19G CARBOHYDRATE 24G, OF WHICH SUGARS 6.6G

FAT 2.1G, OF WHICH SATURATES 0.3G KCALS 197

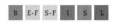

Seared Lamb Salad with Beans & Garlic Mint Dressing

1 garlic clove, crushed

zest of 1 lemon

1 tsp ground cumin

1 tbsp olive oil, plus extra
  for searing

500g/1lb 2oz lamb fillet

150g/5½oz green beans, trimmed

250g/9oz mixed green leaves

½ red onion, thinly sliced

150g/5½oz/1 cup cherry
  tomatoes, halved

GARLIC MINT DRESSING

1 bulb of garlic

a drizzle of olive oil

200g/7oz/generous ¾ cup
  Greek yogurt

1 handful of mint leaves

1 tsp xylitol or honey

2 tbsp balsamic vinegar

a pinch of ground cumin

½ tsp Dijon mustard

sea salt and ground black pepper

This light, herby dressing is delicious over a range of meats and is rich in friendly probiotics to support digestive health. If possible, leave the lamb to marinate overnight before cooking. Lamb is an excellent source of iron and zinc, which is important for male and female fertility, as well as the growth of the baby.

1 Mix together the garlic, lemon zest, cumin and olive oil and rub over the lamb. Cover and leave to marinate in the fridge for 2 hours, or overnight.

2 For the dressing, preheat the oven to 180°C/350°F/Gas 4. Put the garlic bulb on a piece of foil and drizzle over a little olive oil. Bake for about 30 minutes. Leave to cool slightly, then squeeze out the garlic flesh into a blender or food processor. Add the remaining dressing ingredients and blend together, then season to taste.

3 Turn the oven up to 220°C/425°F/Gas 7. Heat a little olive oil in a frying pan over a medium heat and sear the lamb so that it is brown all over. Transfer to a baking tin and roast for 15 minutes. Leave to rest for 5 minutes, then thinly slice.

4 Blanch the beans in a saucepan of boiling water until al dente, then drain and refresh under cold water.

5 Pile the green leaves on a serving plate and top with the beans, onion and tomatoes. Top with the lamb and serve drizzled with the dressing.

SERVES: 4 • PREPARATION TIME: 15 MINUTES, PLUS AT LEAST 2 HOURS MARINATING • COOKING TIME: 50 MINUTES
NUTRITIONAL INFORMATION PER SERVING: PROTEIN 29.2G CARBOHYDRATE 7G, OF WHICH SUGARS 6.1G
FAT 26.3G, OF WHICH SATURATES 11.9G KCALS 381

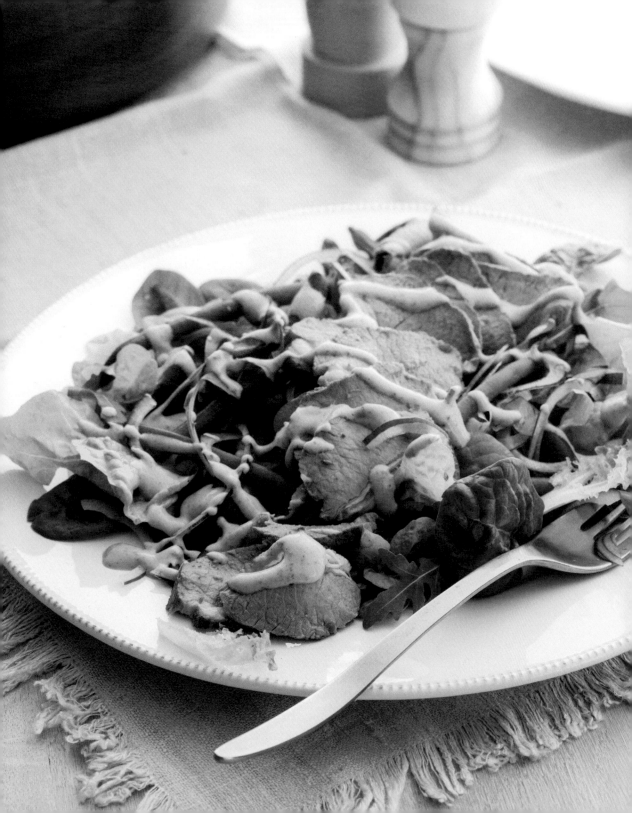

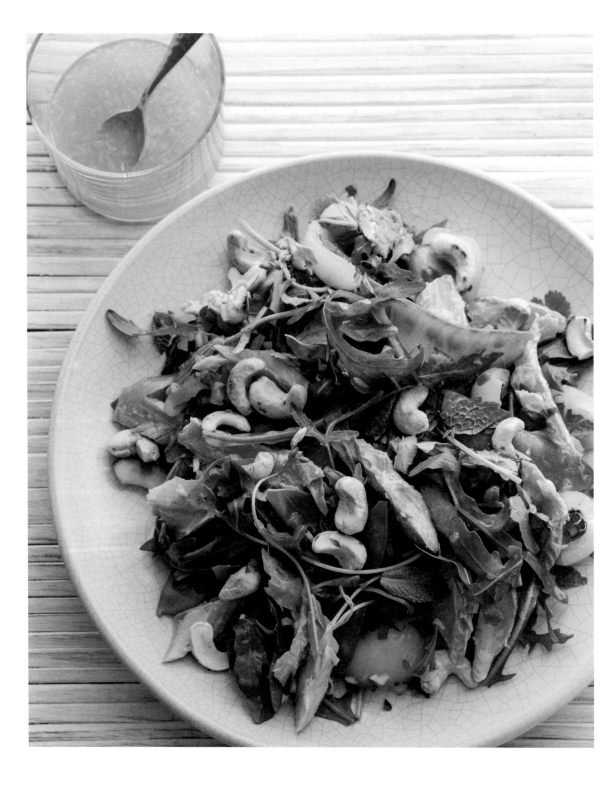

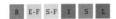

Flaked Trout with Rocket, Lychees & Sweet Lime Dressing

The oily richness of trout contrasts beautifully with the sweet lychees and peppery rocket leaves. Hot-smoked trout requires no preparation, making this a speedy, healthy lunch or evening meal. Trout is an oily fish and a useful source of omega-3 fats. It's also rich in protein and B-vitamins, including niacin, B12 and B6, which are important for ovulation.

60g/2¼oz/heaped ⅓ cup cashew nuts

150g/5½oz mangetout

2 large handfuls of rocket leaves

½ cucumber, halved lengthways, deseeded and sliced

10 lychees, peeled, halved and pitted

1 handful of basil leaves, roughly chopped

1 handful of mint leaves, roughly chopped

1 handful of coriander leaves, roughly chopped

1 red chilli, deseeded and diced

½ red onion, diced

225g/8oz hot-smoked trout

SWEET LIME DRESSING

juice of 2 limes

2 tsp xylitol

1–2 tbsp fish sauce, to taste

1 Lightly toast the cashews in a dry frying pan over a medium heat for about 1 minute, stirring.

2 Blanch the mangetout in a saucepan of boiling water for 30 seconds, then drain and refresh under cold water.

3 Put the mangetout in a serving bowl with the rocket, cucumber, lychees, herbs, chilli and onion and toss together. Break up the trout and scatter over the top of the salad, then sprinkle with the toasted cashews.

4 To make the dressing, mix together the lime juice, xylitol and fish sauce in a non-reactive bowl. Drizzle over the salad and serve.

SERVES: 2 • PREPARATION TIME: 10 MINUTES • COOKING TIME: 2 MINUTES

NUTRITIONAL INFORMATION PER SERVING: PROTEIN 36.6G CARBOHYDRATE 35.8G, OF WHICH SUGARS 30.5G

FAT 20.1G, OF WHICH SATURATES 4G KCALS 449

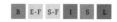

Harissa Sardines with Tahini Yogurt Dressing

A delicious light dish full of Moroccan flavours. Sardines are rich in numerous nutrients that support both male and female fertility, and the addition of lemon and chilli from the harissa makes a wonderful marinade for their rich, oily flesh. Accompany with the creamy tahini yogurt sauce and a salad for a simple, nourishing meal.

juice and zest of 1 lemon

1 tbsp olive oil, plus extra for frying

1 tablespoon harissa paste

4 fresh sardines, scaled, gutted and gills removed

60g/2¼oz/heaped ⅓ cup pine nuts

60g/2¼oz/½ cup pitted black olives, halved

1 handful of coriander leaves, chopped

sea salt and ground black pepper

leafy green salad, to serve

TAHINI YOGURT DRESSING

150g/5½oz/scant ⅔ cup Greek yogurt

3 tbsp tahini

juice of ½ lemon

2 garlic cloves, crushed

a pinch of ground cumin

a pinch of sea salt

1 Mix together all the dressing ingredients in a small non-reactive bowl. Cover and chill until required.

2 Mix together the lemon juice, olive oil and harissa paste in a separate non-reactive dish and leave to one side. Season the sardines with salt and pepper.

3 Heat a griddle pan or frying pan over a medium heat and drizzle over a little olive oil. Add the sardines to the pan and cook for 2–3 minutes. Turn the sardines over, pour over the harissa mixture and cook for a further 2–3 minutes. Add the pine nuts and olives and warm through for 1 minute, then sprinkle over the coriander.

4 Serve the sardines with a leafy green salad and the tahini yogurt dressing.

SERVES: 2 • PREPARATION TIME: 10 MINUTES • COOKING TIME: 7 MINUTES
NUTRITIONAL INFORMATION PER SERVING: PROTEIN 25.7G CARBOHYDRATE 3.2G, OF WHICH SUGARS 2.8G
FAT 32.6G, OF WHICH SATURATES 7G KCALS 410

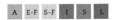

Spinach, Walnut & Roasted Pear Salad with Raspberry Vinaigrette

A simple sweet and tangy salad. Including turmeric adds a wonderful golden glow to the pears and is a fabulous healing spice, too, while goji berries are rich in antioxidants to aid the functioning of the immune system. For additional protein, add a little crumbled feta cheese, if you like.

75g/2½oz/¾ cup walnut halves

1 tbsp butter or coconut butter

1 tsp turmeric

2 tsp honey

2 ripe pears, cored and cut into wedges

200g/7oz baby spinach leaves

1 handful of watercress

1 handful of sprouted beans or seeds, such as alfalfa

1 handful of goji berries

sea salt and ground black pepper

RASPBERRY VINAIGRETTE

4 tbsp raspberry vinegar

2 tbsp balsamic vinegar

1 tsp honey

4 tbsp olive oil

3 tbsp walnut oil

1 tsp Dijon mustard

1 Lightly toast the walnuts in a dry frying pan over a medium heat for about 1 minute, stirring.

2 Heat the butter in a large non-stick frying pan. When the butter is melted, add the turmeric and honey. Add the pear wedges in a single layer and season with a pinch of salt. Cook for about 3 minutes, turning once, until lightly browned, then transfer the pears to a plate.

3 Make the vinaigrette by combining the vinegars and honey in a non-reactive bowl. Slowly whisk in the oils and then the mustard. Season with black pepper.

4 Put the spinach and watercress on a serving plate and scatter over the pears, sprouted beans, toasted walnuts and goji berries. Season with salt and pepper, drizzle over the dressing and serve.

SERVES: 2 • PREPARATION TIME: 10 MINUTES • COOKING TIME: 4 MINUTES
NUTRITIONAL INFORMATION PER SERVING: PROTEIN 8.5G CARBOHYDRATE 34.9G, OF WHICH SUGARS 33.3G
FAT 44.1G, OF WHICH SATURATES 6.2G KCALS 573

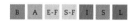

Avocado, Orange & Sea Vegetable Salad with Sprouted Seeds

This simple vibrant salad is easy to assemble and delicious served on its own as a light meal or as an accompaniment to seafood or pan-fried tofu. Sea vegetables are a useful source of iodine required for the production of thyroid hormones, which are important for a woman's hormonal cycle as well as the development of an embryo. Bags of dried sea vegetables are available in most large supermarkets or healthfood shops.

30g/1oz mixed sea vegetables

2 large handfuls of rocket leaves

1 avocado, peeled, pitted and thinly sliced

1 orange, peeled

½ red onion, thinly sliced

1 handful of sprouted seeds, such as alfalfa, mung bean etc

MISO & GINGER DRESSING

1 tbsp white miso paste

½ tsp peeled and grated root ginger

1 tbsp xylitol

3 tbsp mirin

juice of 1 lemon

1 tbsp sesame oil

2 tbsp olive oil

sea salt and ground black pepper

1 Mix all the dressing ingredients together in a non-reactive bowl, season to taste and leave to one side.

2 Soak the sea vegetables in water for 5 minutes, or according to the packet instructions, then drain.

3 Put the rocket in a large bowl with the sea vegetables. Drizzle over a little of the dressing and toss gently. Divide the leaves between two plates and top with the avocado slices. Cut the orange into thin slices, then cut the slices into quarters. Scatter the orange, red onion and sprouted seeds over the salad. Drizzle over the dressing just before serving.

SERVES: 2 • PREPARATION TIME: 10 MINUTES, PLUS 5 MINUTES SOAKING

NUTRITIONAL INFORMATION PER SERVING: PROTEIN 8.6G CARBOHYDRATE 16.6G, OF WHICH SUGARS 13.7G

FAT 24.3G, OF WHICH SATURATES 4.1G KCALS 322

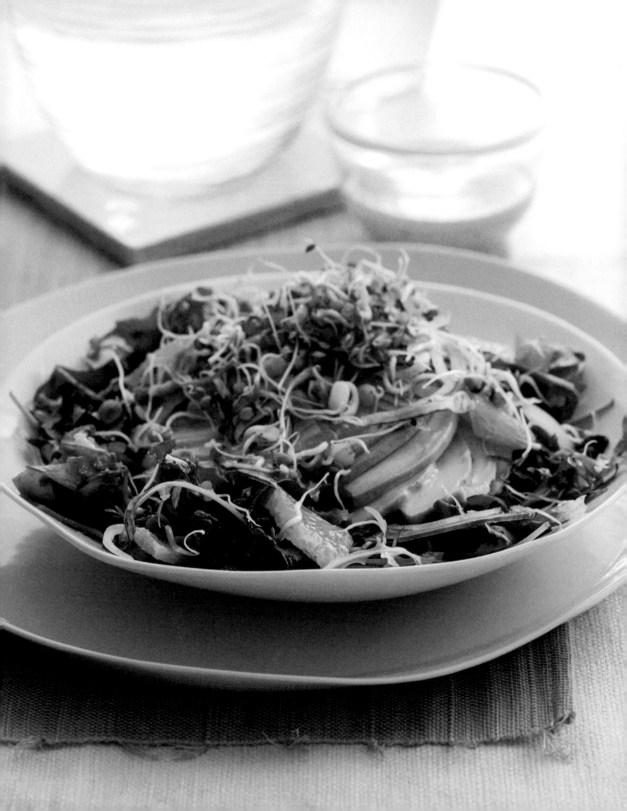

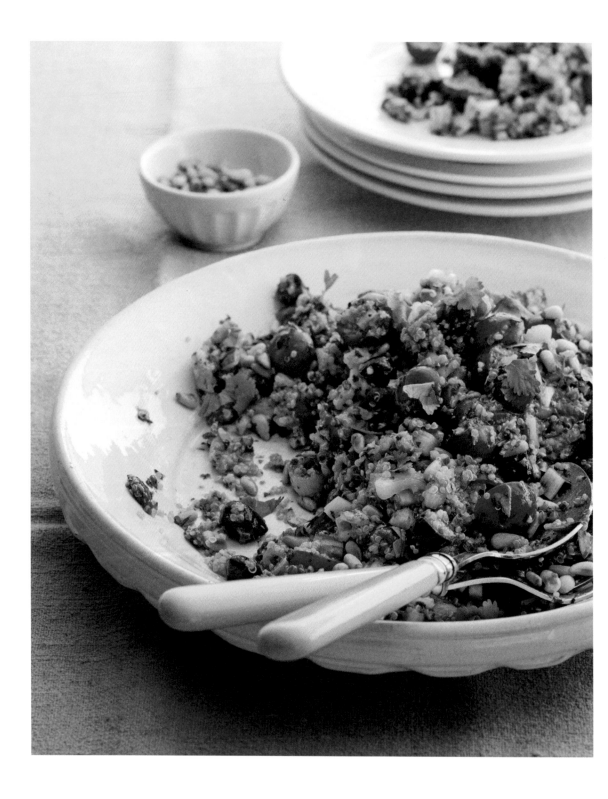

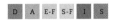

Sicilian Quinoa Bowl

140g/5oz/⅔ cup quinoa

375ml/13fl oz/1½ cups vegetable stock

a pinch of saffron strands

2 jarred roasted red peppers, chopped

2 celery sticks, chopped

60g/2¼oz/½ cup pitted black olives, halved

200g/7oz/1⅓ cups cherry tomatoes, halved

1 small red onion, diced

30g/1oz/scant ¼ cup toasted pine nuts, to serve

coriander leaves, to serve

HERB DRESSING

2 tbsp capers, drained and rinsed

1 anchovy fillet, chopped

1 garlic clove, crushed

1 handful of mint leaves

1 handful of coriander leaves

1 handful of parsley leaves

3 tbsp flaxseed oil

3 tbsp olive oil

3 tbsp red wine vinegar

This wonderful Mediterranean-inspired dish is full of antioxidants, and the quinoa is packed with flavonoids and fibre. It is perfect for packed lunches and delicious warm or cold. Prepare in advance to allow the flavours to develop. For additional protein, serve with sliced roast chicken or prawns, or leave out the anchovy to make it vegetarian.

1 Put the quinoa in a sieve and rinse well. Transfer to a saucepan, pour over the vegetable stock and add the saffron. Bring to the boil over a medium heat, then turn the heat down to low, cover with a lid and leave to simmer for 15 minutes until the quinoa is tender. Remove the pan from the heat, leaving the lid on, and leave the quinoa to steam for a further 5 minutes, then transfer to a serving bowl.

2 To make the dressing, put the capers, anchovy, garlic, herbs, oils and vinegar in a food processor and pulse lightly to combine.

3 Add the peppers, celery, olives, tomatoes and onion to the quinoa and toss everything together. Pour the dressing over the quinoa and toss again to coat. Sprinkle the pine nuts and coriander leaves over the top and serve.

SERVES: 4 • PREPARATION TIME: 15 MINUTES • COOKING TIME: 20 MINUTES
NUTRITIONAL INFORMATION PER SERVING: PROTEIN 8G CARBOHYDRATE 26.5G, OF WHICH SUGARS 9.9G
FAT 31G, OF WHICH SATURATES 3.5G KCALS 428

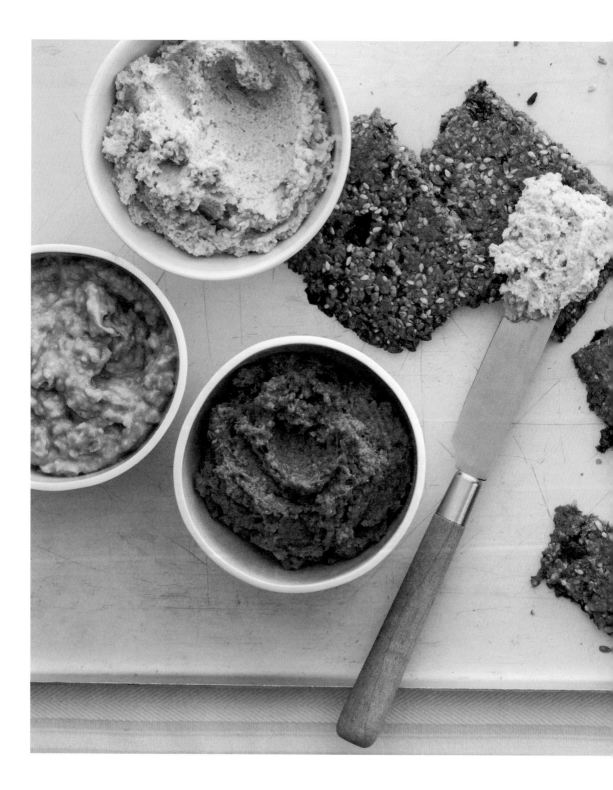

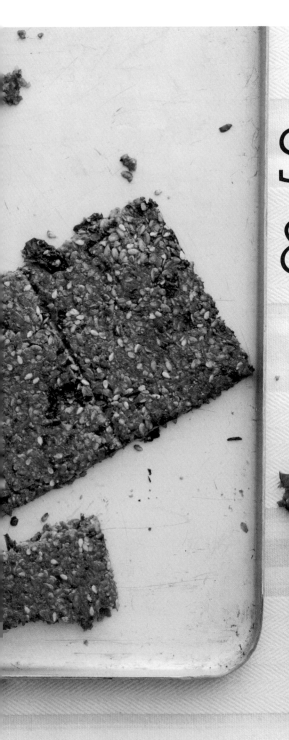
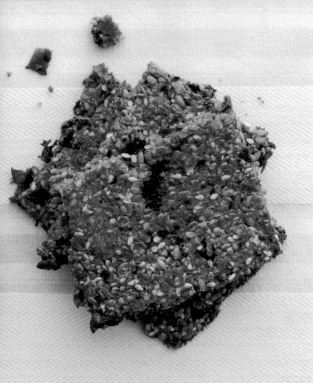

Snacks
& Treats

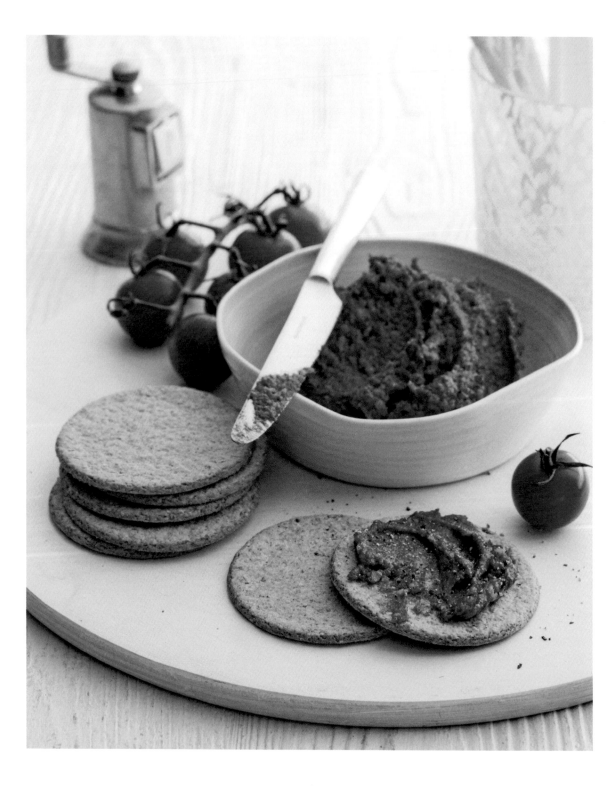

Red Pepper & Tomato Nut Spread

1 garlic clove, crushed
a pinch of paprika
115g/4oz/¾ cup cashew nuts
1 jarred roasted red pepper
6 sundried tomatoes, chopped
1 tbsp nutritional yeast flakes
1 tbsp balsamic vinegar, or to taste
1 tsp xylitol or honey
sea salt and ground black pepper

1 Put the garlic, paprika, cashews, red pepper and tomatoes in a food processor and process until finely chopped.
2 Add the remaining ingredients and blend until smooth. Adjust the quantity of vinegar according to taste. Season lightly with salt and pepper and serve.

SERVES: 4 • PREPARATION TIME: 5 MINUTES
NUTRITIONAL INFORMATION PER SERVING: PROTEIN 7.8G CARBOHYDRATE 10.6G, OF WHICH SUGARS 5.2G FAT 18G, OF WHICH SATURATES 3.3G KCALS 235

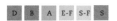

Roasted Aubergine & Mint Dip

1 aubergine
1 tbsp olive oil
1 small red onion, finely diced
1 garlic clove, finely chopped
1 tbsp lemon juice
a pinch of dried chilli flakes
a pinch of smoked paprika
½ tsp ground cumin
1 handful of mint leaves, chopped
sea salt and ground black pepper

1 Preheat the oven to 180°C/350°F/Gas 4. Prick the aubergine skin and place it on a baking tray. Roast for 30–40 minutes until the flesh is soft. Remove from the oven and leave to cool. Peel away the skin and scoop out the flesh into a food processor.
2 Heat the oil in a frying pan over a medium heat and sauté the onion and garlic for 5 minutes until softened. Add them to the food processor with the remaining ingredients. Pulse to combine, but leave some texture. Season to taste, then serve.

SERVES: 4 • PREPARATION TIME: 10 MINUTES • COOKING TIME: 45 MINUTES
NUTRITIONAL INFORMATION PER SERVING: PROTEIN 0.9G CARBOHYDRATE 2.3G, OF WHICH SUGARS 1.6G FAT 2.7G, OF WHICH SATURATES 0.4G KCALS 35

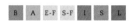

Wasabi Guacamole

This Asian-flavoured guacamole is simple to throw together and fabulous served with vegetables or topped on oat cakes and crackers. Avocado is one of the important foods for fertility, helping both men and women.

1 avocado, peeled and pitted

2 spring onions, finely chopped

a squeeze of lemon juice

¼ tsp wasabi paste

2 tsp soy sauce

2 tsp mirin

1 Put the avocado and spring onions in a bowl and mash gently together. Mix in the remaining ingredients and mash to combine but keep some texture, then serve.

SERVES: 4 • PREPARATION TIME: 5 MINUTES
NUTRITIONAL INFORMATION PER SERVING: PROTEIN 0.7 CARBOHYDRATE 1G,
OF WHICH SUGARS 0.6G FAT 4.9G, OF WHICH SATURATES 1G KCALS 51

Indian-Spiced Onion Hummus

1 tbsp olive oil, plus extra to serve

1 small red onion, thinly sliced

1 tsp xylitol

400g/14oz tinned chickpeas, drained and rinsed

juice of ½ lemon

2 tbsp tahini

1 tsp ground cumin

a pinch of turmeric

1 garlic clove, crushed

1 tsp sea salt

1 Heat the oil in a frying pan and sauté the onion with the xylitol for about 10 minutes until soft and lightly browned. Remove from the heat and leave to cool.

2 In a food processor, blitz together the chickpeas, lemon juice, tahini, spices, garlic, salt and the cooled onion until smooth. Tip into a serving bowl, drizzle with a little olive oil and serve.

SERVES: 4 • PREPARATION TIME: 10 MINUTES • COOKING TIME: 10 MINUTES
NUTRITIONAL INFORMATION PER SERVING: PROTEIN 6.8G CARBOHYDRATE 10.8G,
OF WHICH SUGARS 1.2G FAT 10.2G, OF WHICH SATURATES 1.4G KCALS 159

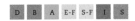

Mixed Seed Crackers

Enjoy these crackers with any of the dips. They are gluten-free and packed with healthy fats. The addition of nori provides essential minerals, including iodine, and the hemp seeds provide an excellent source of protein and are packed with healthy omega-3 fats. They also contain plenty of disease-fighting, plant-based phytonutrients and protective antioxidants such as vitamin E. These will keep in an airtight container for up to 1 week.

½ red pepper, deseeded and chopped

75g/2½oz/scant ⅔ cup sunflower seeds

150g/5½oz/1 cup flaxseeds

1 tomato, chopped

60g/2¼oz/½ cup sundried tomatoes

2 tbsp sesame seeds

2 tbsp hemp seeds

1 nori sheet, crumbled

1 tsp sea salt

1 tsp ground cumin

1 tsp ground coriander

a pinch of cayenne pepper

1 garlic clove, crushed

juice of ½ lemon

1 Preheat the oven to 150°C/300°F/Gas 2. Line a baking tray with baking parchment or a Teflex sheet.

2 Put the red pepper, sunflower seeds and flaxseeds in a food processor and process to break up. Add the remaining ingredients and process again to combine.

3 Spread the mixture onto the prepared baking tray. Shape into a rectangle and mark out 16 squares by gently scoring the surface with a knife. Bake for 30 minutes until golden and crisp. Leave to cool on the baking tray, then break the rectangle into crackers by snapping along the scored lines.

Pictured on page 96 with Red Pepper & Tomato Nut Spread, Wasabi Guacamole and Indian-Spiced Onion Hummus

Makes: 16 crackers • Preparation time: 10 minutes • Cooking time: 30 minutes
Nutritional information per cracker: Protein 4g Carbohydrate 4.3g, of which sugars 0.8g
Fat 10.1g, of which saturates 1.2g Kcals 121

Sweet Curried Cashew Nuts

2 tbsp maple syrup

1 tsp garam masala

1 tsp lemon juice

½ tsp sea salt

150g/5½oz/1 cup cashew nuts

1 Preheat the oven to 150°C/300°F/Gas 2 and line a baking tray with baking parchment.

2 In a bowl, mix together all the ingredients except the cashews. Add the nuts and toss thoroughly to coat, then spread over the prepared baking tray. Bake for 10–15 minutes, stirring occasionally and being careful not to let them brown too much. Leave to cool before serving.

SERVES: 6 • PREPARATION TIME: 5 MINUTES • COOKING TIME: 15 MINUTES
NUTRITIONAL INFORMATION PER SERVING: PROTEIN 4.5G CARBOHYDRATE 7.5G,
OF WHICH SUGARS 4G FAT 10.1G, OF WHICH SATURATES 2.4G KCALS 158

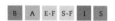

Tangy Tomato Kale Crisps

6 sundried tomatoes

70g/2½oz/heaped ½ cup sunflower seeds

1½ tablespoons nutritional yeast flakes

1 red pepper, deseeded and chopped

1 garlic clove, peeled

1 shallot

2 tbsp balsamic vinegar

2 tbsp filtered water

½ tsp sea salt

a pinch of smoked paprika

250g/9oz kale, chopped

1 Put the tomatoes in a bowl, cover with water and leave to soak for 30 minutes, then drain. Preheat the oven to 150°C/300°F/ Gas 2 and line a baking tray with baking parchment.

2 Put all the ingredients except the kale into a food processor and blend together until smooth. Pour over the kale and mix well, massaging in with your hands to make sure it is all coated.

3 Spread the kale onto the prepared baking tray and bake for 15–20 minutes. Carefully turn them over and cook for a further 5 minutes. You could also dry them in a dehydrator for 10 hours.

SERVES: 6 • PREPARATION TIME: 10 MINUTES, PLUS 30 MINUTES SOAKING
• COOKING TIME: 25 MINUTES
NUTRITIONAL INFORMATION PER SERVING: PROTEIN 5.4G CARBOHYDRATE 5.1G,
OF WHICH SUGARS 2G FAT 8.9G, OF WHICH SATURATES 1.2G KCALS 124

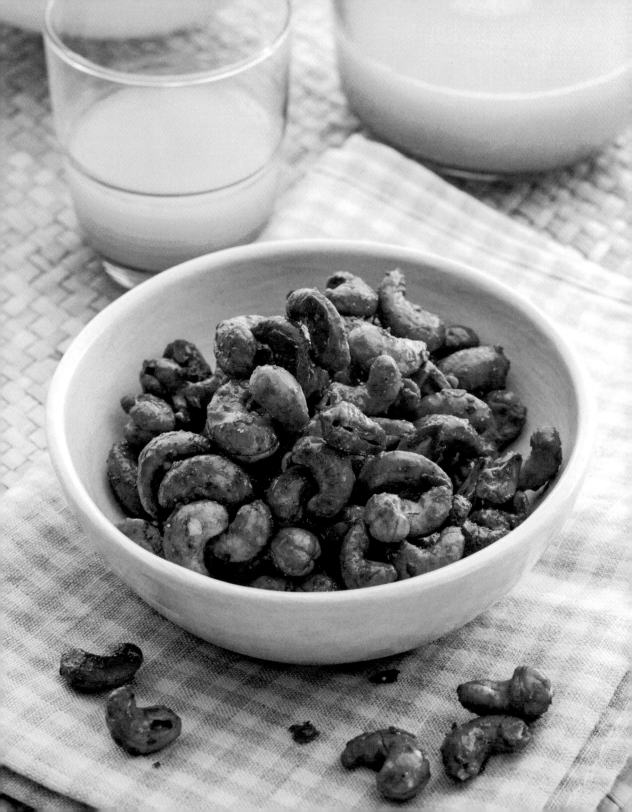

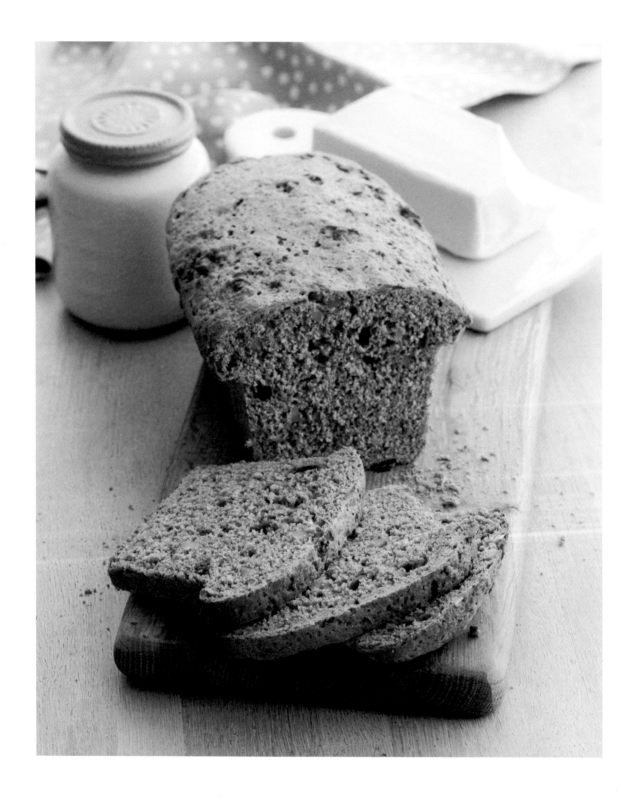

Walnut & Raisin Spelt Bread

This delicious light, nutty bread is wonderful toasted and spread with a little butter or nut butter. Spelt flour is lower in gluten than many other flours, making it lighter on the digestive system. Walnuts are a great source of thiamin and vitamin B6 as well as folic acid, which is critical to preventing birth defects in babies. They're also an excellent source of minerals, such as manganese, copper and magnesium.

350g/12oz/2¾ cups spelt flour, plus extra for dusting

7g/¼oz dried fast-acting yeast

1 tsp caster sugar

1 tsp salt

2 tbsp olive oil

225ml/7¾fl oz/scant 1 cup lukewarm full-fat milk

60g/2¼oz/⅔ cup walnuts, chopped

30g/1oz/¼ cup raisins

1 Put the flour, yeast, sugar and salt into a food processor and mix thoroughly. Combine the oil and warm milk in a jug and, with the food processor running slowly, pour into the flour mixture to make a soft dough. Pulse in the walnuts and raisins. Turn out the dough onto a work surface and knead for 5 minutes.

2 Put the dough in a clean bowl, cover with cling film and leave in a warm place to rise for 1–1½ hours until the dough has doubled in volume.

3 Turn the dough out onto a lightly floured surface and knead well with the palm of your hand for 2–3 minutes. Transfer the dough to a 450g/1lb loaf tin and leave to rise again for 30 minutes.

4 Preheat the oven to 220°C/425°F/Gas 7. Bake the bread for 20–25 minutes, or until golden and it sounds hollow when you tap your knuckles on the bottom. Leave to cool on a wire rack.

MAKES: 1 LOAF (10 SLICES) • PREPARATION TIME: 15 MINUTES, PLUS 2 HOURS PROVING • COOKING TIME: 25 MINUTES
NUTRITIONAL INFORMATION PER SLICE: PROTEIN 6.4G CARBOHYDRATE 24.4, OF WHICH SUGARS 4.4G
FAT 7.6G, OF WHICH SATURATES 1.3G KCALS 192

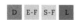

Courgette Chocolate Brownies

These grain-free brownies are packed with protein and healthy fats thanks to the addition of the nut butter and almonds. No one would ever know they also contain courgettes. Low in sugar, this is a rich and indulgent treat. Pecan nuts are little nuggets of nutrition – they are rich in many phytochemicals and antioxidants which can help protect the body's cells and DNA from damage as well as support immune health.

200g/7oz/heaped ¾ cup almond butter

200g/7oz dark chocolate, 70% cocoa solids, broken into pieces

100g/3½oz/½ cup xylitol

3 eggs

1 tsp vanilla extract

60g/2¼oz/heaped ½ cup ground almonds

1 tsp ground cinnamon

1 tsp bicarbonate of soda

1 courgette, about 125g/4½oz, finely grated

60g/2¼oz/½ cup chopped pecan nuts (optional)

1 Preheat the oven to 180°C/350°F/Gas 4. Grease and line a square 20cm/8in baking tin with baking parchment.

2 Put the nut butter, chocolate and xylitol in a saucepan over a low heat and warm gently to melt the chocolate. Transfer the mixture to a food processor, add the eggs, vanilla extract, ground almonds, cinnamon and bicarbonate of soda and process to combine. Process in the courgette, then stir in the chopped pecans, if using. Spoon the mixture into the prepared baking tin.

3 Bake for 20–25 minutes until firm to touch. Leave to cool in the tin, then cut into 16 squares.

MAKES: 16 BROWNIES • PREPARATION TIME: 10 MINUTES • COOKING TIME: 25 MINUTES
NUTRITIONAL INFORMATION PER BROWNIE: PROTEIN 5.2G CARBOHYDRATE 15.9G, OF WHICH SUGARS 14.1G
FAT 17.5G, OF WHICH SATURATES 13.5G KCALS 225

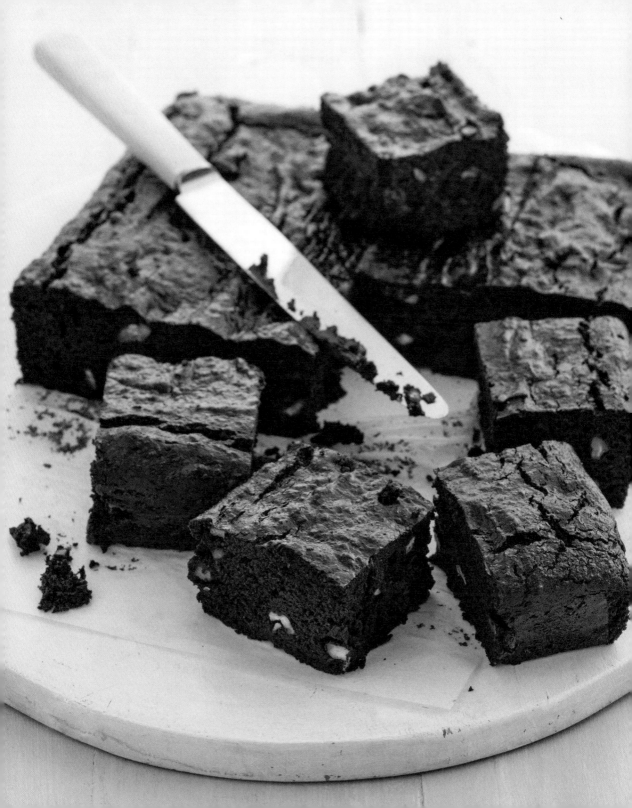

Molasses Ginger Cookies

180g/6¼oz/1½ cups almond flour

¼ tsp sea salt

½ tsp bicarbonate of soda

1 teaspoon ground ginger

1 tsp peeled and grated root
ginger

½ tsp ground cinnamon

60g/2¼oz/¼ cup coconut butter

1 tbsp molasses

2 tbsp honey

1 Preheat the oven to 180°C/350°F/Gas 4 and line a baking tray
with baking parchment.

2 Combine the dry ingredients in a large bowl. In a smaller bowl,
stir together the wet ingredients, then mix them into the dry
ingredients until well incorporated.

3 Spoon 10 balls of the mixture onto the prepared baking tray,
spacing them a little way apart, and gently press to flatten them
into circles. Bake for 7–10 minutes until crisp. Leave to cool on
the baking tray.

MAKES: 10 COOKIES • PREPARATION TIME: 10 MINUTES • COOKING TIME: 10 MINUTES
NUTRITIONAL INFORMATION PER COOKIE: PROTEIN 3.8G CARBOHYDRATE 5.6G, OF WHICH
SUGARS 5.1G FAT 16.1G, OF WHICH SATURATES 6G KCALS 182

Figs Dipped in Chocolate

100g/3½oz dark chocolate, 75%
cocoa solids, broken into pieces

4 figs, quartered

60g/2¼oz/½ cup finely chopped
pistachio nuts

1 Put the chocolate in a heatproof bowl and rest it over a pan of
simmering water, making sure the bottom of the bowl does not
touch the water. Heat, stirring, until the chocolate has melted.

2 Lay a piece of baking parchment on a tray. Dip a fig quarter into
the melted chocolate so that it reaches halfway up, then dip
it into the chopped nuts. Put on the tray and repeat with the
remaining fig quarters. Store in the fridge until ready to eat.

SERVES: 2–4 • PREPARATION TIME: 10 MINUTES • COOKING TIME: 5 MINUTES
NUTRITIONAL INFORMATION PER FIG: PROTEIN 4.3G CARBOHYDRATE 18.6G,
OF WHICH SUGARS 18.4G FAT 15.4G, OF WHICH SATURATES 5.3G KCALS 231

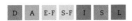

Superfood Truffles

These little chocolate nuggets are packed with superfoods designed to nourish and energize the body. Mulberries are a superfruit high in antioxidants, which help scavenge free radicals from the body and that also provide a boost to circulation. They are a great energizing fruit, rich in natural sugars and iron as well as B-vitamins needed for the production of energy.

30g/1oz/⅓ cup goji berries

115g/4oz/scant ½ cup cashew or almond butter

60g/2¼oz/¼ cup maple syrup

2 tbsp cacao powder, or to taste

60g/2¼oz cacao butter or dark chocolate, melted

2 tsp maca powder

a pinch of sea salt

½ tsp vanilla extract

1 tsp super-green powder, such as wheatgrass

1 tsp ground cinnamon

30g/1oz/scant ⅓ cup shelled hemp seeds

30g/1oz/¼ cup mulberries or dried cherries

shredded coconut, cacao powder or crushed pistachio nuts, to decorate

1 Put the goji berries in a bowl, cover with water and leave to soak for 30 minutes, then drain.

2 Put the cashew nut butter, maple syrup, cacao powder and melted cacao butter in a food processor and blitz to combine. Add the remaining ingredients and process to form a dough. Chill in the fridge for about 4 hours or overnight until firm. Alternatively, place in a freezer to firm up.

3 Use a spoon to scoop out the mixture and roll into 16 walnut-sized balls. Roll the balls in a little shredded coconut, crushed pistachios or cacao powder, to decorate, then place on a sheet of baking parchment to set.

MAKES: 16 TRUFFLES • PREPARATION TIME: 10 MINUTES, PLUS 30 MINUTES SOAKING AND AT LEAST 4 HOURS CHILLING

NUTRITIONAL INFORMATION PER TRUFFLE: PROTEIN 2.6 CARBOHYDRATE 6.8G, OF WHICH SUGARS 3.9G

FAT 7.7G, OF WHICH SATURATES 1.6G KCALS 102

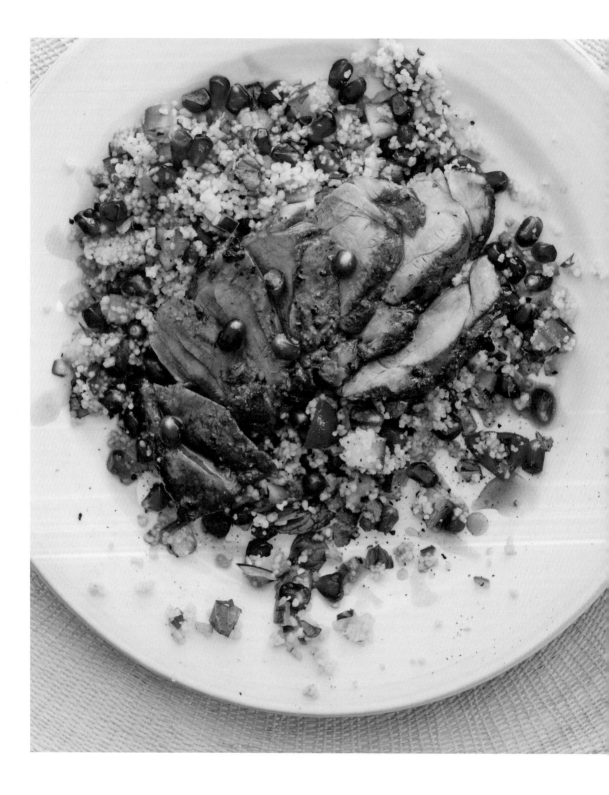

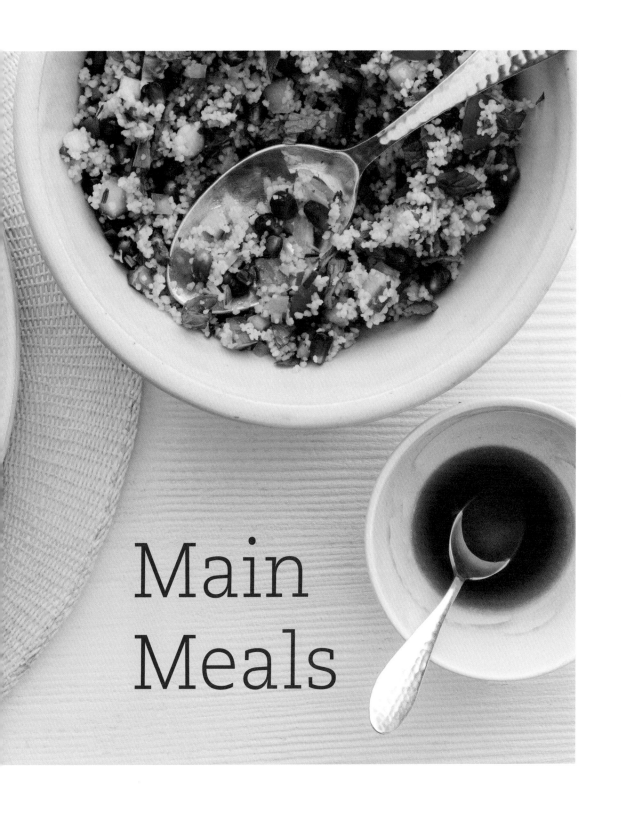

Main Meals

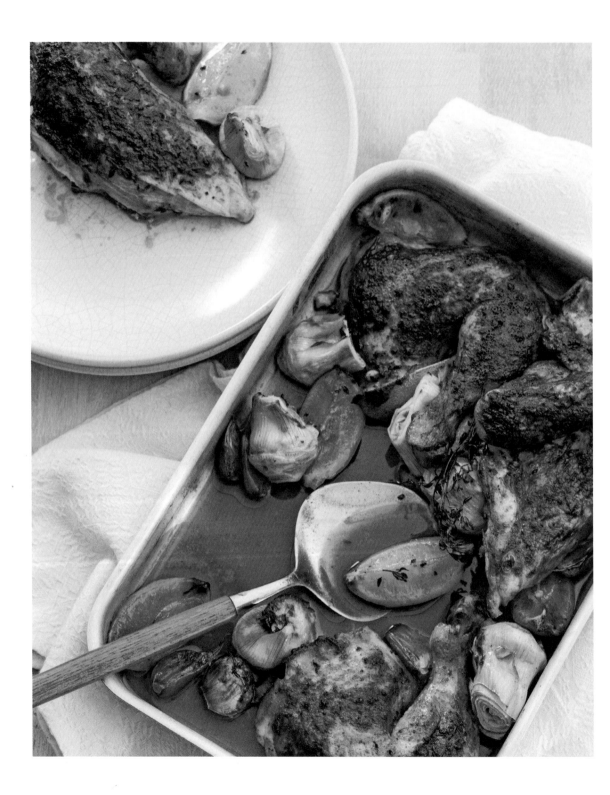

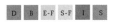

Slow-Roasted Paprika Chicken with Lemon & Artichokes

This is such an easy recipe. Everything is simply placed in a roasting pan and slow cooked in the oven, creating an amazing spicy, lemony flavour. Serve leftovers cold for lunch the next day with salad. Globe artichokes are an excellent source of dietary fibre, magnesium and the trace mineral chromium, which is important for balancing blood sugar.

1 tbsp smoked paprika

1 tsp sumac

3 tbsp olive oil

1 organic chicken, jointed

1 bulb of garlic, separated into unpeeled cloves

2 lemons, quartered

1 sprig of thyme

150ml/5fl oz/scant ⅔ cup chicken stock

400g/14oz tinned artichoke hearts, drained

ground black pepper

1 Preheat the oven to 160°C/315°F/Gas 2–3.

2 Mix together the paprika, sumac and olive oil in a small bowl. Put the chicken pieces in a roasting tin and add the garlic cloves, lemon quarters and thyme. Pour over the paprika oil and rub it all over the chicken pieces. Drizzle over the stock and season with pepper. Cover the roasting tin with foil and roast for 2 hours.

3 Remove the foil from the roasting tin, add the artichoke hearts and turn up the oven to 200°C/400°F/Gas 6. Roast for a further 30 minutes until the chicken is golden and cooked through, then serve.

SERVES: 6 • PREPARATION TIME: 10 MINUTES • COOKING TIME: 2 HOURS 30 MINUTES
NUTRITIONAL INFORMATION PER SERVING: PROTEIN 33.2G CARBOHYDRATE 1.4G, OF WHICH SUGARS 0.6G
FAT 27.8G, OF WHICH SATURATES 7G KCALS 387

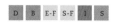

Indonesian Chicken with Buckwheat Noodles

1 lemongrass stalk, chopped

1 handful of coriander leaves

1 small onion, chopped

2 garlic cloves, crushed

2cm/¾in piece root ginger, peeled and grated

1 tbsp coconut sugar or honey

1 tbsp soy sauce

1 tbsp fish sauce

½ tsp turmeric

1 tsp garam masala

400ml/14fl oz/generous 1½ cups coconut milk

4 skinless boneless chicken thighs, cut into large chunks

125g/4½oz buckwheat noodles

1 tsp sesame oil

1 tbsp coconut oil

1 red chilli, deseeded and diced

1 pak choi, cut into strips

100g/3½oz mangetout

4 shiitake mushrooms, sliced

sea salt and ground black pepper

1 handful of bean sprouts, to serve

2 spring onions, chopped, to serve

A hearty meal in a bowl, lightly spiced and packed with nutrient-rich vegetables. This dish contains a wealth of anti-inflammatory ingredients, including ginger, garlic and turmeric, together with immune-supporting shiitake mushrooms and coconut. Buckwheat noodles, also called soba, are a nutritious staple in Asian dishes and provide plenty of slow-release carbohydrates to keep you energized throughout the day.

1 Put the lemongrass, coriander, onion, garlic, ginger, coconut sugar, soy sauce, fish sauce, turmeric, garam masala and coconut milk in a blender or food processor and process until smooth. Pour over the chicken pieces and season lightly with salt and pepper. Cover and leave to marinate in the fridge for at least 2 hours, or overnight.

2 Cook the buckwheat noodles with the sesame oil according to the packet instructions, then drain and refresh under cold water.

3 Meanwhile, heat the coconut oil in a wok or large frying pan. Drain the chicken, reserving the marinade, and stir-fry for 2–3 minutes. Add the chilli, pak choi, mangetout and mushrooms and cook for a further 1 minute. Add the reserved marinade and simmer for 10–15 minutes until the chicken is cooked through. Toss in the noodles and warm through. Sprinkle over the bean sprouts and spring onions and serve.

SERVES: 2 • PREPARATION TIME: 15 MINUTES, PLUS AT LEAST 2 HOURS MARINATING • COOKING TIME: 20 MINUTES
NUTRITIONAL INFORMATION PER SERVING: PROTEIN 32.3G CARBOHYDRATE 29.2G, OF WHICH SUGARS 24.1G
FAT 16.5G, OF WHICH SATURATES 7G KCALS 394

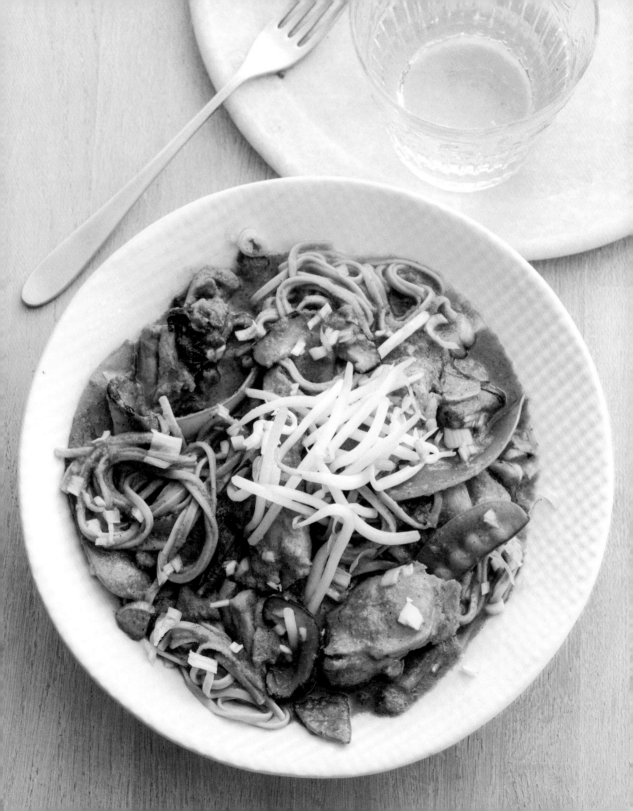

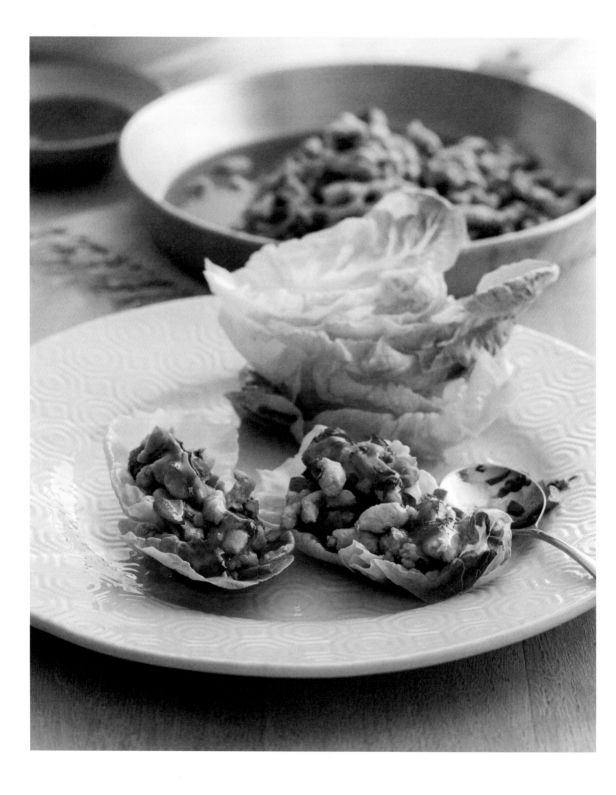

Vietnamese Turkey in Lettuce Wraps

This dish is ideal for an energizing lunch or light evening meal and is so quick and simple to prepare. Spoon the spiced turkey into crisp lettuce leaves and drizzle over a little chilli sauce for an extra kick. A high-protein, low-fat food, turkey is also rich in tryptophan and tyrosine which the body converts to serotonin and dopamine – chemicals that play a role in the production of babymaking hormones.

1 tbsp olive oil

200g/7oz minced turkey

1 small red onion, diced

1 tbsp peeled and grated root ginger

1 red chilli, deseeded and diced

1 handful of coriander leaves, chopped

2 tbsp fish sauce

juice of 1 lime

juice of 1 lemon

1 tbsp honey

1 tbsp soy sauce

sea salt and ground black pepper

2 Little Gem lettuces, leaves separated, to serve

Thai sweet chilli sauce, to serve (optional)

1 Heat the oil in a large frying pan or wok and stir-fry the minced turkey until it begins to turn light brown. Add the onion, ginger and chilli and stir-fry for a further 2–3 minutes. Remove from the heat and stir in the coriander leaves.

2 Combine the fish sauce, lime and lemon juice, honey and soy sauce in a non-reactive bowl. Pour over the turkey and season with salt and pepper to taste.

3 To serve, spoon the mixture into lettuce leaves and drizzle over a little sweet chilli sauce, if you like.

SERVES: 2 • PREPARATION TIME: 10 MINUTES • COOKING TIME: 8 MINUTES
NUTRITIONAL INFORMATION PER SERVING: PROTEIN 26.9G CARBOHYDRATE 13.9G, OF WHICH SUGARS 13.4G
FAT 11G, OF WHICH SATURATES 2.5G KCALS 263

Tamarind-Glazed Duck with Watermelon Salsa

This is a wonderful sweet-and-sour marinade, which is equally delicious on chicken. The refreshing watermelon salsa is the perfect foil for the rich tamarind duck. Tamarind is high in dietary fibre, which aids digestion and helps to stabilize blood-sugar levels, while duck is packed with fertility-boosting nutrients, including B-vitamins, selenium and zinc.

2 garlic cloves

1 small onion, cut into wedges

2 tomatoes, halved

1 tbsp olive oil

75g/2½oz/heaped ¼ cup tamarind paste

1 pickled chilli

1 tbsp honey

2 duck breasts

mixed salad leaves, to serve

WATERMELON SALSA

150g/5½oz watermelon, peeled and finely diced

juice of 1 lime

½ red chilli, deseeded and finely chopped

½ red onion, finely chopped

sea salt and ground black pepper

1 Preheat the oven to 200°C/400°F/Gas 6.

2 Put the garlic, onion and tomatoes on a baking tray and drizzle over the olive oil. Bake for 15 minutes until the tomatoes are soft. Leave to cool slightly.

3 Put the roasted garlic, tomatoes and onion in a blender or food processor with the tamarind paste, chilli and honey and purée until smooth. Score the skin of the duck breasts, then pour the sauce over the duck and leave to marinate for at least 30 minutes.

4 Heat a griddle or large frying pan over a medium heat. Drain the duck breasts, reserving the marinade, then sear, skin side down. Turn the heat down to low and cook for about 10 minutes until the fat has rendered. Transfer the duck to a shallow roasting tin and pour over the reserved marinade. Bake for 10 minutes, basting occasionally. Remove from the oven and leave to rest for 10 minutes, then thinly slice.

5 Mix all the salsa ingredients together and season to taste with salt and pepper. Serve the duck with the salsa and a mixed salad.

SERVES: 2 • PREPARATION TIME: 15 MINUTES, PLUS AT LEAST 30 MINUTES MARINATING • COOKING TIME: 35 MINUTES
NUTRITIONAL INFORMATION PER SERVING: PROTEIN 22.1G CARBOHYDRATE 38.5G, OF WHICH SUGARS 18.2G
FAT 11.6G, OF WHICH SATURATES 2.8G KCALS 353

E-F S-F S

Pomegranate-Glazed Lamb with Herby Couscous

2 tbsp pomegranate molasses

1 tbsp olive oil

2 garlic cloves, crushed

1 tsp ground cumin

2 lamb steaks, about 110g/4oz each

sea salt and ground black pepper

POMEGRANATE DRESSING

2 tbsp pomegranate molasses

3 tbsp olive oil

1 tbsp lemon juice

HERBY COUSCOUS

100g/3½oz/½ cup couscous

juice and zest of 1 lemon

2 tbsp extra virgin olive oil

1 small red onion, diced

½ tsp ground cumin

½ tsp sea salt

½ cucumber, deseeded and diced

2 tomatoes, deseeded and chopped

1 large handful of mint leaves, chopped

1 large handful of parsley leaves, chopped

1 preserved lemon, rind only, diced

seeds of 1 pomegranate

Pomegranate molasses creates a delicious sweet, tangy marinade for lamb. Ideally, marinate the meat overnight to let the flavours fully develop. The herby couscous makes a wonderful accompaniment and takes just minutes to prepare.

1 In a bowl, mix together the pomegranate molasses, olive oil, garlic, cumin and salt and pepper, then rub over the lamb steaks. Cover and leave to marinate in the fridge for at least 1 hour, or overnight.

2 Combine the ingredients for the pomegranate dressing in a separate non-reactive bowl and leave to one side.

3 Soak the couscous in 125ml/4fl oz/½ cup boiling water in a large bowl. Cover the bowl with cling film and leave to stand for 10 minutes. Add the remaining couscous ingredients and fluff up with a fork.

4 Meanwhile, preheat the grill until hot, then grill the lamb steaks for about 10–12 minutes, brushing with the marinade occasionally and turning once during cooking to make sure both sides are cooked.

5 Thinly slice the lamb and serve on top of the couscous, drizzled with the pomegranate dressing.

Pictured on page 110

SERVES: 2 • PREPARATION TIME: 15 MINUTES, PLUS AT LEAST 1 HOUR MARINATING • COOKING TIME: 12 MINUTES

NUTRITIONAL INFORMATION PER SERVING: PROTEIN 33.6G CARBOHYDRATE 60.1G, OF WHICH SUGARS 28G

FAT 32.3G, OF WHICH SATURATES 6.9G KCALS 578

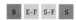

Sensational Spaghetti Bolognese

This family favourite is packed with an array of veggies to boost the nutrient content and served with wholewheat spaghetti for slow-release energy. Instead of lamb you could use turkey mince for a lower fat option. Need to support your immune health? Try shiitake mushrooms, which are rich in polysaccharides, including beta glucans that are shown to boost immune cells.

1 tbsp olive oil

200g/7oz minced lamb

1 onion, finely chopped

2 garlic cloves, finely chopped

1 small carrot, finely chopped

½ red pepper, deseeded and chopped

½ green pepper, deseeded and chopped

1 celery stalk, finely chopped

4 shiitake mushrooms, chopped

2 bay leaves

100ml/3½fl oz/generous ⅓ cup full-fat milk

400g/14oz/scant 1⅔ cups tinned chopped tomatoes

200ml/7fl oz/scant 1 cup vegetable or beef stock

1 tsp thyme leaves, chopped

1 tsp parsley leaves, chopped

1 tsp oregano leaves, chopped

200g/7oz wholewheat spaghetti

2 tbsp grated Parmesan cheese, to serve (optional)

1 Heat the oil in a large casserole pan over a high heat and fry the minced lamb until browned. Add the onion and garlic and fry gently for 1–2 minutes, or until softened. Add the carrot, peppers, celery, mushrooms and bay leaves to the pan and cook for a further 1 minute.

2 Add the milk, tomatoes and stock to the pan and bring to the boil. Turn the heat down and leave to simmer for 1 hour until the sauce has thickened and the mince is tender, then stir in the herbs.

3 Meanwhile, cook the spaghetti according to the packet instructions.

4 To serve, pile the spaghetti onto plates and top each with the Bolognese sauce and grated Parmesan, if you like.

SERVES: 4 • PREPARATION TIME: 10 MINUTES • COOKING TIME: 1 HOUR 10 MINUTES
NUTRITIONAL INFORMATION PER SERVING: PROTEIN 24.1G CARBOHYDRATE 18G, OF WHICH SUGARS 7.4G
FAT 17.4G, OF WHICH SATURATES 7.3G KCALS 323

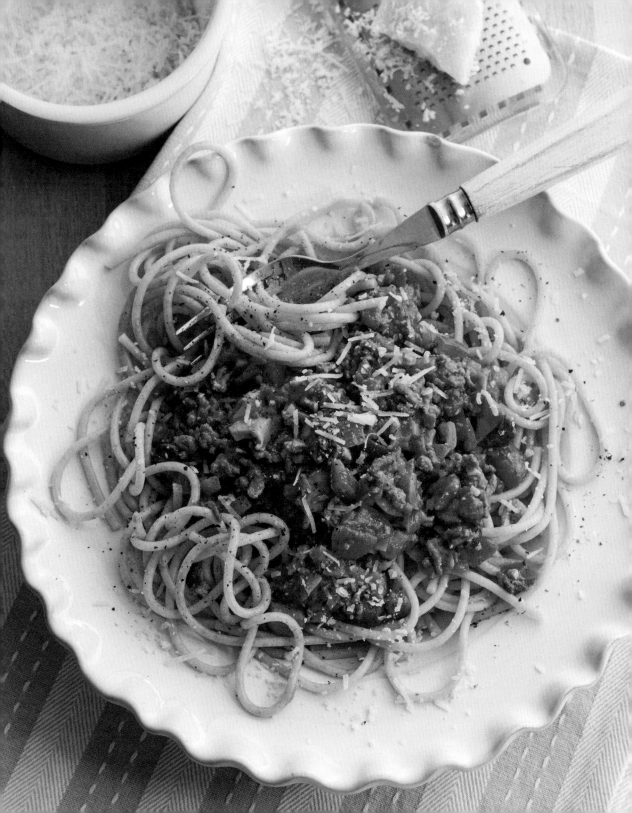

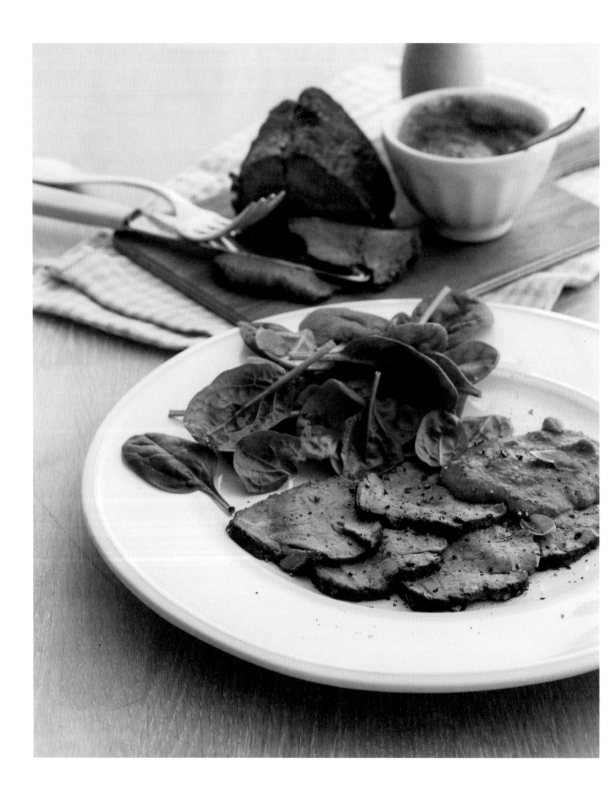

Roast Beef Fillet with Roasted Garlic, Tomato & Herb Sauce

Succulent beef served with a rich, tangy garlic and herb sauce makes a sensational feast. Choose organic beef as it is richer in nutrients.

1 tsp ground cumin

2 garlic cloves, crushed

2 tbsp olive oil

500g/1lb 2oz beef fillet (in one piece)

baby spinach leaves, to serve

ROASTED GARLIC, TOMATO & HERB SAUCE

1 bulb of garlic

1 tbsp olive oil, plus extra for drizzling

1 shallot, diced

250g/9oz/1⅔ cups cherry tomatoes

4 anchovy fillets

1 tsp xylitol or caster sugar

1 tbsp balsamic vinegar

25g/1oz/scant ¼ cup sultanas

1 tbsp capers, drained and rinsed

50g/1¾ oz/⅓ cup blanched almonds

4 tbsp extra virgin olive oil

100ml/3½fl oz/generous ⅓ cup passata

1 small bunch of parsley, chopped

1 small bunch of basil, leaves picked

sea salt and ground black pepper

1 Mix the cumin, crushed garlic and the 2 tablespoons olive oil together and rub all over the beef fillet. Cover and leave to marinate in the fridge for at least 2 hours, or overnight.

2 For the sauce, preheat the oven to 180°C/350°F/Gas 4. Slice off the top quarter of the garlic bulb. Put the bulb on a piece of foil, drizzle over a little olive oil and season. Wrap up in the foil and roast for 40 minutes. Leave the garlic to cool slightly, then squeeze the roasted flesh out of the bulb into a food processor, discarding the skin. Turn up the oven to 200°C/400°F/Gas 6.

3 Heat the 1 tablespoon oil in a frying pan over a medium heat and sauté the shallot, tomatoes and anchovy fillets with the sugar and vinegar. Cook for 5 minutes, then add to the food processor with the garlic and all the remaining sauce ingredients, except the herbs. Blend to form a thick sauce, adding a little water to thin the sauce slightly, if necessary. Transfer to a saucepan and add the parsley and basil.

4 Remove the beef from the marinade. Heat a heavy-based frying pan and sear the beef on all sides. Place the fillet in a roasting tin and roast for 20 minutes until cooked through. Leave to rest for 10 minutes before carving.

5 Heat the sauce and spoon over the beef. Serve with a baby-leaf spinach salad.

SERVES: 4 • PREPARATION TIME: 15 MINUTES, PLUS AT LEAST 2 HOURS MARINATING • COOKING TIME: 1 HOUR 5 MINUTES
NUTRITIONAL INFORMATION PER SERVING: PROTEIN 31.3G CARBOHYDRATE 9.6G, OF WHICH SUGARS 8.6G,
FAT 31G, OF WHICH SATURATES 6.4G KCALS 442

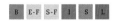

Chilli-Glazed Salmon with Cucumber Lime Salad

In this dish, fillets of wild Alaskan salmon are marinated in a tangy Asian-style dressing and accompanied by a light and refreshing cucumber salad. Salmon is an excellent source of omega-3 fatty acids, which are important for circulation and male and female fertility.

1 pickled chilli, drained

2 garlic cloves, crushed

1 tbsp soy sauce

2 tbsp apple cider vinegar

2 tbsp coconut sugar or xylitol

2 boneless wild Alaskan salmon fillets, with skin

CUCUMBER LIME SALAD

2 tbsp lime juice

1 tbsp xylitol

1 tbsp mirin

1 handful of bean sprouts

1 cucumber, halved and thinly sliced

2 spring onions, sliced finely

1 tbsp chopped cashew nuts

1 small handful of mint leaves, chopped

1 small handful of coriander leaves, chopped

1 Put the chilli, garlic, soy sauce, vinegar and coconut sugar in a food processor and process to combine. Put the salmon fillets in a shallow, non-reactive dish. Pour over the marinade, cover and leave to marinate in the fridge for 30 minutes.

2 Make the dressing for the salad by mixing together the lime juice, xylitol and mirin in a small bowl until the xylitol has dissolved. Put the bean sprouts, cucumber, spring onions, cashews, mint and coriander in another bowl, pour over the dressing and toss until well combined.

3 Preheat the grill to high and line a baking tray with foil. Remove the salmon from the marinade, reserving the marinade, and place on the prepared baking tray. Grill for about 7 minutes, or until the fish is golden and just cooked through.

4 Meanwhile, put the reserved marinade in a small saucepan and simmer to reduce slightly to form a thicker, sticky glaze. Pour over the cooked salmon and serve with the cucumber lime salad.

SERVES: 2 • PREPARATION TIME: 10 MINUTES, PLUS 30 MINUTES MARINATING • COOKING TIME: 7 MINUTES
NUTRITIONAL INFORMATION PER SERVING: PROTEIN 23.4G CARBOHYDRATE 26.9G, OF WHICH SUGARS 24.4G
FAT 14.9G, OF WHICH SATURATES 2.6G KCALS 305

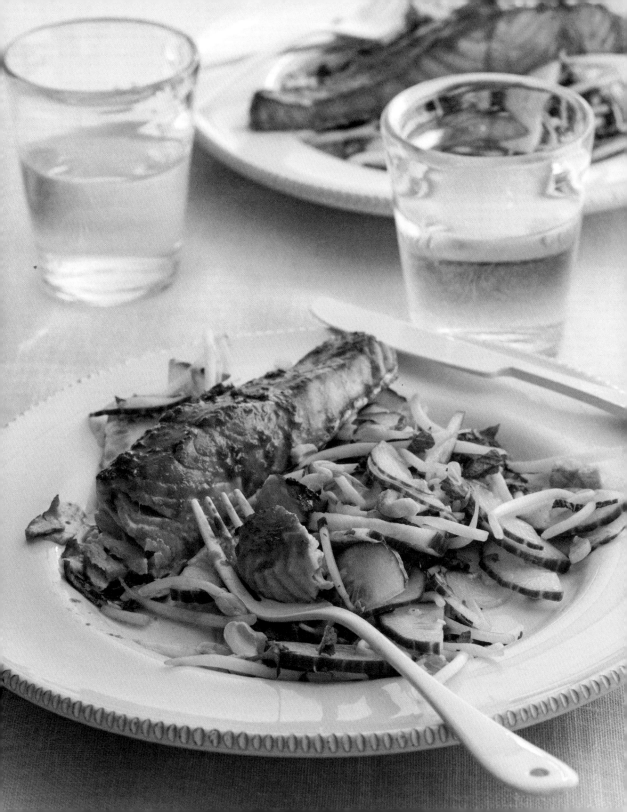

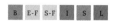

Baked Sea Bass with Salsa Verde

Baking fish in parcels keeps the flesh wonderfully moist and the salsa verde infuses the fish with an amazing aroma of fresh herbs. This makes a simple yet delicious light meal. Accompany with salad and new potatoes, if you like. Sea bass is an excellent source of high-quality protein, B-vitamins and omega-3 fatty acids and minerals such as selenium and magnesium, which is an important anti-stress mineral.

2 skinless sea bass fillets, about 130g/4½oz each

1 lemon, sliced

sea salt and ground black pepper

SALSA VERDE

1 bunch of parsley leaves

1 bunch of basil leaves

1 handful of mint leaves

2 garlic cloves, crushed

2 anchovy fillets

2 tbsp capers, drained and rinsed

2 tbsp red wine vinegar

1 tsp Dijon mustard

½ red onion, diced

75ml/2¼fl oz/scant ⅓ cup olive oil, plus extra for drizzling

1 Preheat the oven to 200°C/400°F/Gas 6.

2 Put all the ingredients for the salsa verde except the oil in a food processor and pulse until the mixture is roughly chopped. Gradually add the oil and pulse to combine. Season with salt and pepper.

3 Lay out two square sheets of baking parchment, each large enough to wrap around a fish fillet. Drizzle the paper with a little oil and top with the fish fillets. Season with salt and pepper and lay over a couple of the lemon slices. Place a spoonful of the salsa verde on top of each fillet, reserving the remaining salsa. Wrap up each fish parcel, tucking the ends under. You can secure the parcels in foil, if you like.

4 Transfer the parcels to a baking tray and bake for 12–15 minutes until just cooked. Serve the fish with the reserved salsa verde.

SERVES: 2 • PREPARATION TIME: 10 MINUTES • COOKING TIME: 15 MINUTES
NUTRITIONAL INFORMATION PER SERVING: PROTEIN 20.8G CARBOHYDRATE 1.9G, OF WHICH SUGARS 1G
FAT 40.5G, OF WHICH SATURATES 5.8G KCALS 458

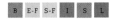

Pan-Fried Halibut with Caramelized Balsamic Onions

Sweet caramelized onions make a delicious accompaniment to the light soft flesh of halibut. You can prepare the onions in advance and reheat when ready to cook the fish. Halibut is truly a nutrient-dense food; it is high in protein, B-vitamins and tryptophan, which is useful for boosting mood and may help to boost libido.

juice and zest of 1 lemon

2 tbsp olive oil, plus extra for frying

1 tbsp chopped rosemary

2 halibut fillets, skin on

sea salt and ground black pepper

CARAMELIZED ONION SAUCE

1 tbsp coconut oil

2 large onions, sliced

1 tsp chopped rosemary

1 garlic clove, crushed

400g/14oz/scant 1⅔ cups tinned chopped tomatoes

2 tbsp red wine vinegar

30g/1oz/¼ cup raisins

zest of 1 lemon

juice of ½ lemon

1 tsp xylitol or honey

1 handful of parsley leaves, chopped

1 Combine the lemon juice and zest, olive oil and 1 tablespoon chopped rosemary in a shallow non-reactive dish and season with salt and pepper. Add the halibut fillets and turn to coat. Cover and leave to marinate for 1 hour.

2 To make the sauce, heat the coconut oil in a saucepan over a low heat and fry the onions with the rosemary and garlic very gently for 15 minutes. Add the remaining sauce ingredients and cook for a further 15 minutes.

3 When ready to serve, heat a little olive oil in a frying pan over a medium heat. Pan-fry the halibut for about 3–4 minutes on each side, or until cooked through. Serve with the onion sauce.

SERVES: 2 • PREPARATION TIME: 15 MINUTES, PLUS 1 HOUR MARINATING • COOKING TIME: 1 HOUR 5 MINUTES
NUTRITIONAL INFORMATION PER SERVING: PROTEIN 24.5G CARBOHYDRATE 21.1G, OF WHICH SUGARS 20G
FAT 15.8G, OF WHICH SATURATES 5.5G KCALS 324

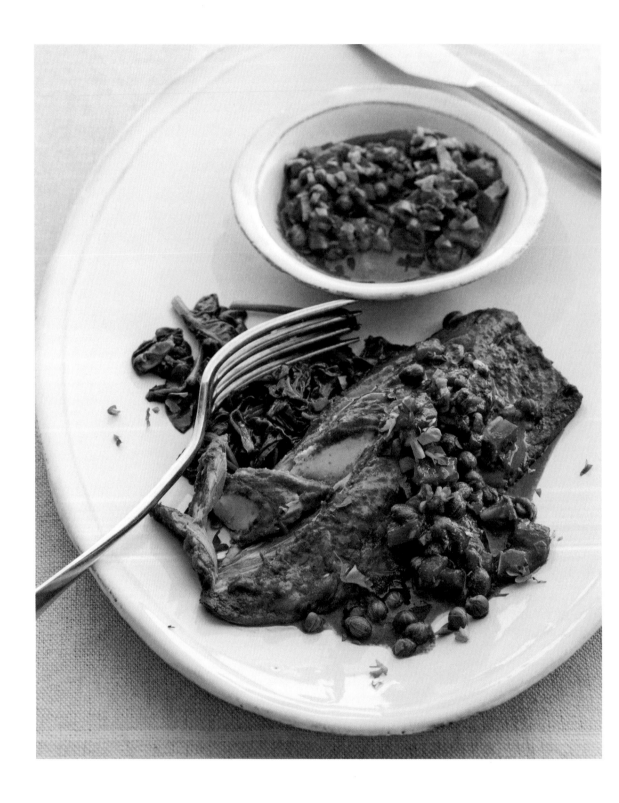

Moroccan-Spiced Mackerel

This recipe is full of North African flavours. The tangy marinade is rich in anti-inflammatory spices and makes a delicious dressing to serve over the cooked fish. For an extra nutrient boost, sprinkle with pine nuts – they are a good source of vitamin E, which has been shown to increase fertility when given to both men and women. Serve with a simple chickpea salad or steamed leafy greens.

2 mackerel fillets, skin on

1 jarred roasted red pepper, chopped

1 tbsp capers, drained and rinsed

1 handful of parsley leaves, chopped

1 preserved lemon, rind only, finely chopped

2 spring onions, finely chopped

1 tablespoon toasted pine nuts (optional)

MARINADE

6 tbsp olive oil

4 tbsp red wine vinegar

2 tbsp sweet smoked paprika

1 tsp turmeric

2 tsp ground cumin

4 garlic cloves, crushed

sea salt and ground black pepper

1 Mix all the marinade ingredients together in a small non-reactive bowl. Put the mackerel fillets in a shallow non-reactive dish and spoon over half of the marinade. Cover and leave to marinate in the fridge for 30 minutes.

2 To make the dressing, add the red pepper, capers, parsley, preserved lemon and spring onions to the remaining marinade.

3 Preheat the grill to medium-high and line a baking tray with foil. Put the marinated mackerel fillets on the prepared baking tray and grill for 5 minutes until cooked through.

4 Serve the mackerel drizzled with the dressing. Scatter over a few pine nuts, if you like.

SERVES: 2 • PREPARATION TIME: 10 MINUTES, PLUS 30 MINUTES MARINATING • COOKING TIME: 5 MINUTES
NUTRITIONAL INFORMATION PER SERVING: PROTEIN 23.9G CARBOHYDRATE 6.8G, OF WHICH SUGARS 5.9G
FAT 45.9G, OF WHICH SATURATES 7.2G KCALS 535

Prawn Skewers with Sweet Tomato Chutney

Succulent prawns flavoured with garlic and chilli and served with a tangy tomato chutney makes a delicious, energizing dish. The chutney can be prepared ahead and will keep in the fridge for several days. It can be used as an accompaniment to meat and fish dishes and is wonderful with goats' cheese. Accompany with a mixed salad. Lack of certain nutrients such as zinc can affect a man's fertility. Prawns are a good source of zinc as well as selenium and cholesterol, required for the production of testosterone.

2 tbsp olive oil
1 garlic clove, crushed
1 pickled chilli, finely chopped
juice and zest of 1 lime
12 raw, peeled king prawns
sea salt and ground black pepper
mixed salad, to serve

SWEET TOMATO CHUTNEY
1 tbsp olive oil
1 garlic clove, crushed
2 tsp peeled and grated root ginger
1 shallot, finely chopped
3 tbsp apple cider vinegar
400g/14oz/scant 1⅔ cups tinned chopped tomatoes
a pinch of ground cinnamon
a pinch of ground cloves
2 tbsp xylitol

1 To make the chutney, heat the oil in a saucepan over a medium heat and sauté the garlic and ginger for 1 minute. Add the remaining ingredients and bring the mixture to the boil. Turn the heat down and leave to simmer for 30 minutes until the mixture is thick and sticky, stirring occasionally to prevent it burning. Leave to cool. Meanwhile, soak 4 wooden skewers in water.

2 Mix together the oil, garlic, chilli and lime zest and juice and season. Put the prawns in a shallow non-reactive dish. Pour over the marinade, cover and leave to marinate in the fridge for 15 minutes.

3 Preheat the grill to high. Thread 3 prawns onto each skewer, put them on a baking tray and drizzle over any remaining marinade. Grill for 2–3 minutes, or until the prawns just turn pink, turning halfway through cooking. Serve the skewers with the sweet tomato chutney and a mixed salad.

SERVES: 2 • PREPARATION TIME: 15 MINUTES, PLUS 15 MINUTES MARINATING • COOKING TIME: 35 MINUTES
NUTRITIONAL INFORMATION PER SERVING: PROTEIN 7.8G CARBOHYDRATE 22.2G, OF WHICH SUGARS 20.7G
FAT 13.9G, OF WHICH SATURATES 2G KCALS 227

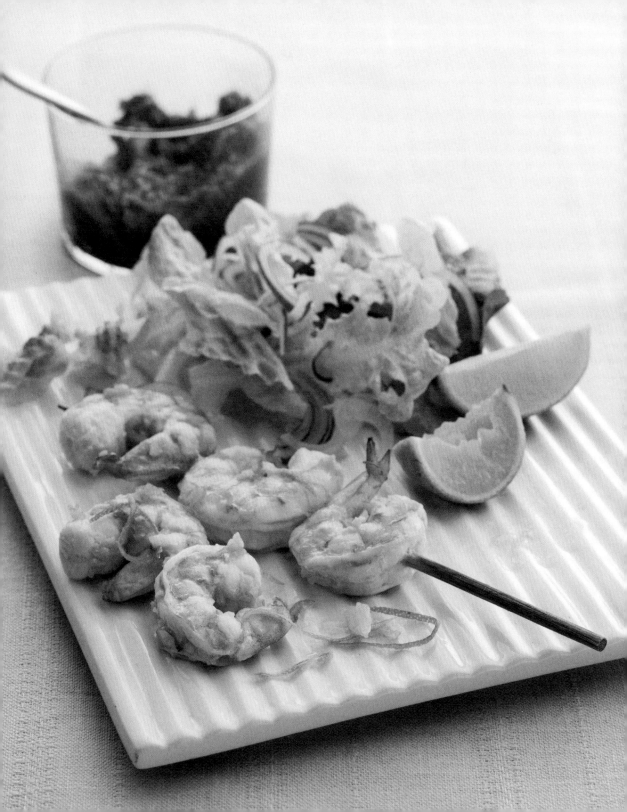

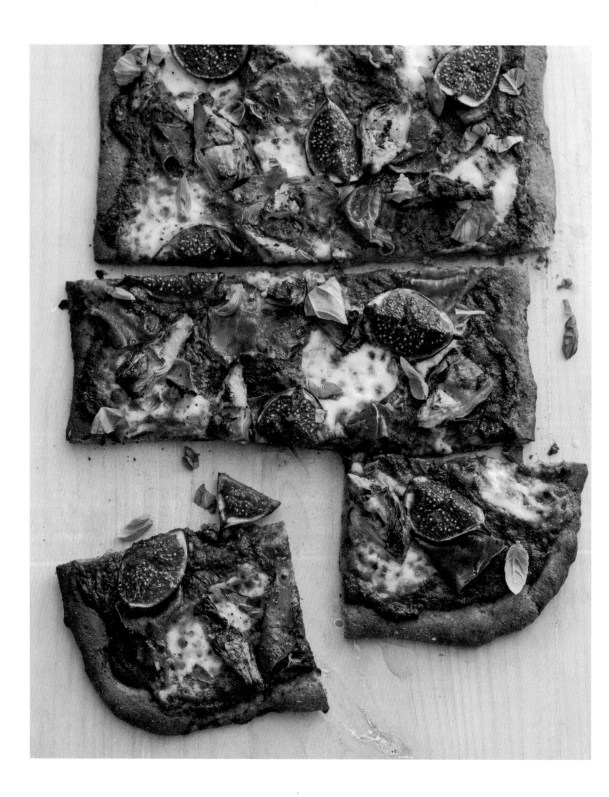

Fertility Pizza

PIZZA BASE

100ml/3½fl oz/⅓ cup plus 2 tbsp warm milk

7g/¼oz dried fast-acting yeast

200g/7oz/1⅔ cups spelt flour

1 tsp sea salt

1 tbsp olive oil, plus extra for greasing

polenta, for dusting

TOMATO SAUCE

200ml/7fl oz/scant 1 cup passata

4 sundried tomatoes

a pinch of dried chilli flakes

1 garlic clove, crushed

a pinch of xylitol (optional)

2 tbsp chopped basil leaves

sea salt and ground black pepper

TOPPING

2 cooked artichoke hearts, thinly sliced

150g/5½oz buffalo mozzarella cheese, sliced

4 slices of prosciutto or Parma ham, ripped up into bite-sized pieces

2 figs, quartered

a drizzle of olive oil

1 handful of basil leaves, to serve

Who says you can't have a healthy pizza? This version is packed with an array of fertility-boosting foods on a delicious spelt base – perfect for when you want a carb fix. Spelt is an ancient grain with a deep nutty flavour. It is rich in soluble fibre, manganese and magnesium, and protein, making it an ideal energizing grain.

1 Pour the milk into a jug and sprinkle over the yeast. Leave to stand for 5 minutes. Put the flour, salt and oil in a large bowl and add the milk mixture. Stir well to form a dough. Knead well for 5 minutes. Alternatively, use a mixer and process for 5 minutes.

2 Coat the inside of a bowl with a little olive oil, put the dough in the bowl and cover with cling film. Leave it to rise in a warm place for 1 hour.

3 Make the tomato sauce by putting all the ingredients in a food processor and blending until smooth.

4 Preheat the oven to 220°C/425°F/Gas 7. Sprinkle a baking sheet with a little polenta. Turn the dough out onto the baking sheet and roll out the dough to form a rectangle or round.

5 Spread the tomato sauce over the dough base, leaving a 2.5cm/1in border. Top with the artichokes, mozzarella, prosciutto and figs. Drizzle the pizza with oil and season with salt and pepper. Bake for 15–20 minutes, or until the bread is crisp and golden brown and the cheese has melted. Scatter basil over the top of the pizza and serve.

SERVES: 2 • PREPARATION TIME: 20 MINUTES, PLUS 1 HOUR PROVING • COOKING TIME: 20 MINUTES
NUTRITIONAL INFORMATION PER SERVING: PROTEIN 18.7G CARBOHYDRATE 64.7G, OF WHICH SUGARS 4.9G
FAT 9.8G, OF WHICH SATURATES 2.5G KCALS 422

Chipotle-Spiced Tofu Wraps

This smoky chilli tomato sauce adds a wonderful flavour to tofu while cooking. Vary the toppings in the wraps according to taste – try salsa, shredded lettuce or avocado. Tempeh could also be used instead of tofu in this protein-packed dish. Any leftover tofu can be served with a salad for a light, nutritious meal. Chilli peppers increase blood flow to the reproductive system and organs as well as the rest of the body. They also help to stimulate endorphins, which helps to relieve stress that can be a contributing factor in infertility.

1 dried chipotle chilli

4 plum tomatoes, halved

3 garlic cloves

3 tbsp olive oil

1 handful of coriander leaves, chopped

250g/9oz firm tofu

½ red onion, chopped

2 flour tortillas

sea salt and ground black pepper

Mango & Coriander Salsa (see page 85), to serve

shredded lettuce leaves and slices of avocado, to serve (optional)

1 Soak the chilli in warm water for 20 minutes, then drain.

2 Preheat the grill to medium-high. Put the tomatoes and garlic in a flameproof baking dish. Drizzle over 1 tablespoon of the olive oil and grill for 15 minutes until the tomatoes are lightly golden. Put the tomatoes and garlic in a food processor with the chilli, coriander and salt and pepper and pulse to form a coarse purée.

3 Slice the tofu into thick slices and season with salt and pepper.

4 Heat 1 tablespoon of the oil in a frying pan over a medium heat. Add the onion and sauté for 2–3 minutes, then remove from the pan. Heat the remaining oil and pan-fry the tofu for about 2–3 minutes on each side until golden. Add the tomato purée and onion and cook for about 3–5 minutes to thicken.

5 Spoon some of the tofu mixture in the centre of each tortilla and top with salsa, lettuce and/or avocado slices, if using. Fold the sides of the wrap over before rolling up. Serve immediately.

SERVES: 2 • PREPARATION TIME: 10 MINUTES, PLUS 20 MINUTES SOAKING • COOKING TIME: 30 MINUTES
NUTRITIONAL INFORMATION PER SERVING: PROTEIN 13.9G CARBOHYDRATE 30.7G, OF WHICH SUGARS 18.6G
FAT 6.2G, OF WHICH SATURATES 0.9G KCALS 234

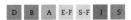

Nut & Seed Falafels with Mint Yogurt

60g/2¼oz/½ cup pumpkin seeds

30g/1oz/¼ cup sunflower seeds

30g/1oz/⅓ cup ground flaxseed

60g/2¼oz/heaped ½ cup cashew nuts

2 tbsp chopped parsley leaves

2 tsp ras el hanout

1 tsp ground cumin

1 small carrot

60g/2¼oz/heaped ⅓ cup sundried tomatoes, chopped

3 tbsp chopped coriander leaves

1 garlic clove, crushed

½ red onion, chopped

30g/1oz/¼ cup pitted black olives

1 tbsp lemon juice

1 tbsp tahini

olive oil, for brushing

sea salt and ground black pepper

Little Gem lettuces, to serve

MINT YOGURT

100g/3½oz/generous ⅓ cup Greek yogurt

juice of ½ lemon

1 garlic clove, crushed

¼ cucumber, peeled, deseeded and finely chopped

zest of 1 lemon

½ tsp sea salt

1 tbsp chopped mint leaves

These Mediterranean-flavoured nuggets are delicious served hot with salad but are also perfect cold in pitta with salad for a healthy meal on the go. The falafels will keep in the fridge for 2–3 days and can be frozen, too. Pumpkin seeds are an excellent source of minerals, especially zinc, which is important for male fertility.

1 Put the pumpkin and sunflower seeds in a small bowl, cover with water and leave to soak for 30 minutes, then drain.

2 For the dressing, mix all the ingredients together in a small non-reactive bowl, season with pepper and chill until required.

3 To make the falafels, put all the seeds and cashews in a food processor and pulse to chop. Add the remaining falafel ingredients, season with salt and pepper and process to combine. Form the mixture into small balls.

4 Preheat the oven to 200°C/400°F/Gas 6 and line a baking tray with foil. Put the falafels on the prepared baking tray, brush them with a little olive oil and bake for 20 minutes until golden. Serve with the yogurt and lettuce leaves.

SERVES: 4 • PREPARATION TIME: 15 MINUTES, PLUS 30 MINUTES SOAKING • COOKING TIME: 20 MINUTES

NUTRITIONAL INFORMATION PER SERVING: PROTEIN 12.8G CARBOHYDRATE 12.3G, OF WHICH SUGARS 4.5G

FAT 35.2G, OF WHICH SATURATES 6.3G KCALS 412

Lemony Pea & Asparagus Red Rice Risotto

A delicious, comforting dish. Red rice has a wonderful nutty flavour and makes a healthier option to white refined rice. Red rice is rich in anthocyanins, antioxidants that can help protect the body's cells from damage. It also contains plenty of soluble fibre, making it useful for supporting energy levels.

1 tbsp olive oil

1 tbsp butter

1 red onion, finely chopped

2 garlic cloves, crushed

125g/4½oz Camargue red rice

500ml/17fl oz/2 cups hot vegetable stock

zest of 1 lemon

1 tbsp lemon juice

150g/5½oz/1 cup frozen peas

1 bunch of asparagus, about 200g/7oz, cut into 2cm/¾in pieces

2 tbsp grated Parmesan cheese

1 Heat the oil and butter in a large shallow saucepan over a medium heat and sauté the onion and garlic for 5 minutes. Add the rice and stir to coat in the oil, then add the vegetable stock. Bring to the boil, then turn the heat down, cover with a lid and leave to simmer for 40 minutes, stirring occasionally, until the rice is almost cooked.

2 Add the lemon zest and juice, peas and asparagus and cook for a further 3–4 minutes until the vegetables and rice are tender.

3 Serve the risotto sprinkled with grated Parmesan.

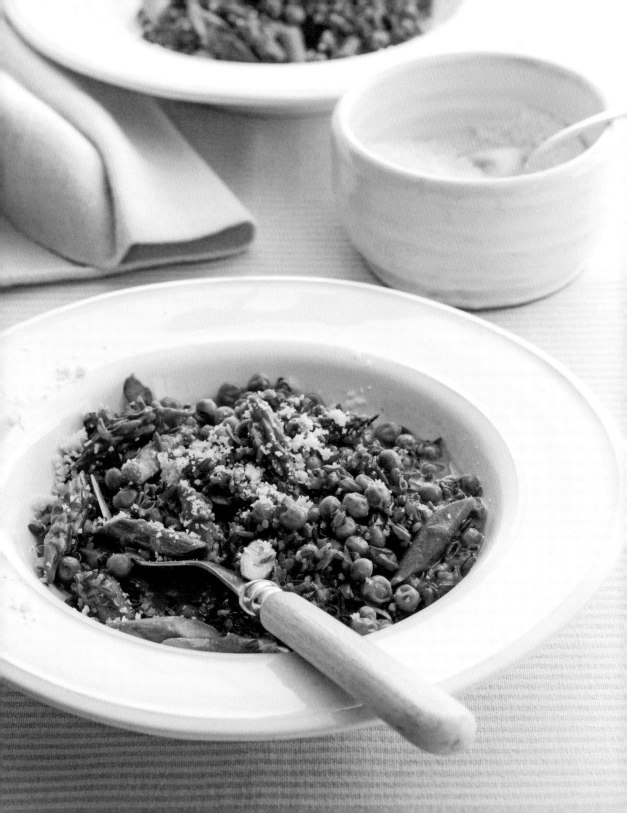

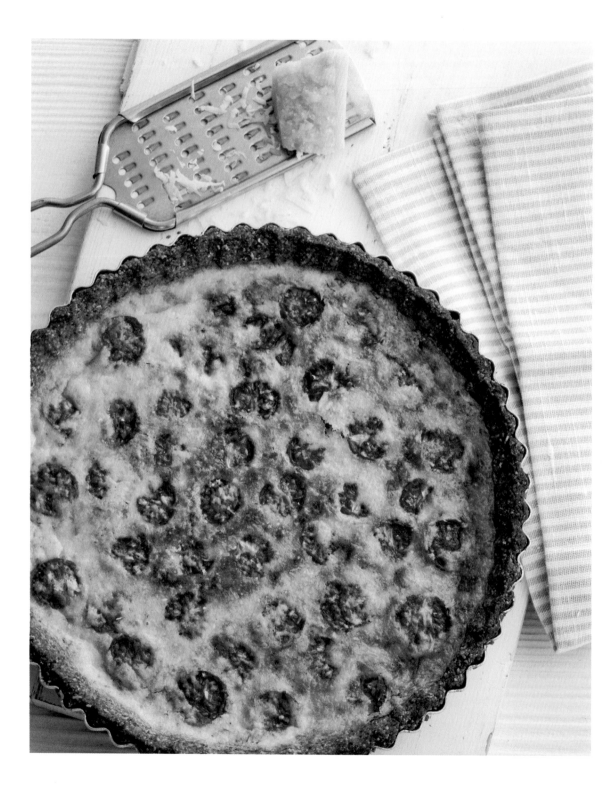

Roasted Tomato & Garlic Almond Tart

Made with a protein-rich almond pastry, this tart is topped with roasted tomatoes scented with garlic and creamy Parmesan to make a satisfying vegetarian dish. Eggs are a nutrient-dense food, providing protein and a good source of iodine, which is often low in our diets. Choose organic eggs, which have a higher nutrient content and more omega-3 fats.

180g/6¼oz/scant 1¼ cup almonds

a pinch of sea salt

1 tbsp chopped parsley leaves

1 tbsp grated Parmesan cheese

2 egg yolks

2 tbsp butter

FILLING

150g/5½oz/1 cup cherry
  tomatoes, halved

2 garlic cloves, unpeeled

olive oil, for drizzling

balsamic vinegar, for drizzling

2 eggs

1 tbsp chopped parsley leaves

125ml/4fl oz/½ cup crème fraîche

2 tbsp grated Parmesan cheese

sea salt and ground black pepper

1 Preheat oven to 180°C/350°F/Gas 4. Put the almonds in a food processor and process to form a flour-like mixture. Pulse in the salt, parsley and Parmesan, then add the egg yolks and butter and process to form a dough. Press the dough into a 20cm/8in tart tin. Bake for 20 minutes until just turning lightly golden.

2 Meanwhile, to make the filling, put the tomatoes and garlic in a roasting tin and drizzle over a little oil and vinegar. Roast for 15 minutes until just softening. Remove from the oven but leave the oven on.

3 Remove the peel from the garlic and put the flesh in a food processor with the eggs, parsley and crème fraîche and purée. Season with salt and pepper. Pour the egg mixture into the case and arrange the cherry tomatoes on top. Sprinkle with grated Parmesan and bake for 30 minutes until lightly golden and set.

SERVES: 6 • PREPARATION TIME: 15 MINUTES • COOKING TIME: 1 HOUR 5 MINUTES
NUTRITIONAL INFORMATION PER SERVING: PROTEIN 12.8G CARBOHYDRATE 3.2G, OF WHICH SUGARS 2.4G
FAT 35.7G, OF WHICH SATURATES 12.2G KCALS 385

Quinoa & Feta Burgers with Tomato Relish

80g/2¾oz/heaped ⅓ cup quinoa

2 tsp bouillon powder

2 tbsp olive oil, plus extra for frying the burgers

½ red onion, finely chopped

2 garlic cloves, crushed

1 tsp ground cumin

400g/14oz tinned black beans or kidney beans, drained and rinsed

115g/4oz feta cheese, crumbled

1 tbsp chopped parsley leaves

1 tbsp chopped mint leaves

2 tbsp cornflour

sea salt and ground black pepper

burger buns, to serve (optional)

lettuce leaves and tomato slices, to serve (optional)

TOMATO RELISH

1 small dried chipotle chilli

4 tomatoes, quartered

1 red onion, quartered

1 tbsp olive oil

1 tbsp coriander leaves

2 tsp xylitol

2 tsp balsamic vinegar

A healthy burger – this vegetarian option is rich in protein and the addition of quinoa and feta provides plenty of calcium to support bone health, too.

1 For the relish, soak the chilli in warm water for 20 minutes, then drain. Preheat the oven to 180°C/350°F/Gas 4. Put the tomatoes and onion on a baking tray, drizzle over the oil and roast for 15 minutes until soft. Put in a food processor with the chilli and the remaining relish ingredients and pulse to form a thick, chunky purée. Leave to cool.

2 Put the quinoa in a saucepan with the bouillon powder and 250ml/9fl oz/1 cup water and bring to the boil. Turn the heat down, cover with a lid and leave to simmer for 15 minutes until cooked. Leave to cool slightly, then transfer to a bowl.

3 Heat the olive oil in frying pan. Add the onion, garlic and cumin and cook, stirring, for about 5 minutes. Remove from the heat and add the beans, feta and cooked quinoa and season with salt and pepper. Stir in the herbs and cornflour, then mash with a potato masher to break up the beans. Leave to cool slightly.

4 When the mixture is cool enough to handle, divide it into 4 equal portions and shape into burgers.

5 Heat some oil in large frying pan over a medium-high heat. Add the burgers and cook for about 5–6 minutes, turning halfway through to brown on both sides.

6 Put the patties in burger buns with the lettuce and tomato, if using, or just serve with salad and the relish.

SERVES: 4 • PREPARATION TIME: 20 MINUTES, PLUS 20 MINUTES SOAKING • COOKING TIME: 40 MINUTES
NUTRITIONAL INFORMATION PER SERVING (NO BUN): PROTEIN 8.5G CARBOHYDRATE 24G,
OF WHICH SUGARS 6.2G FAT 9.7G, OF WHICH SATURATES 3.4G KCALS 215

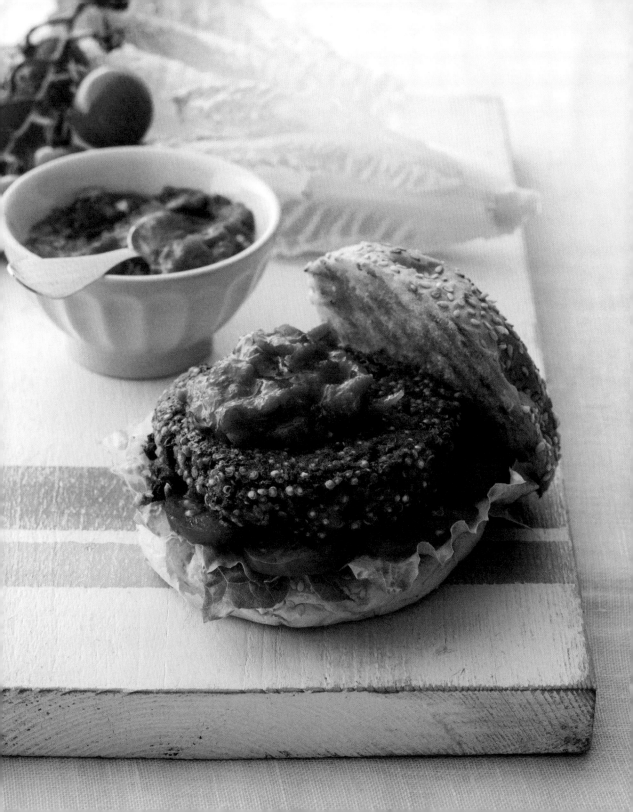

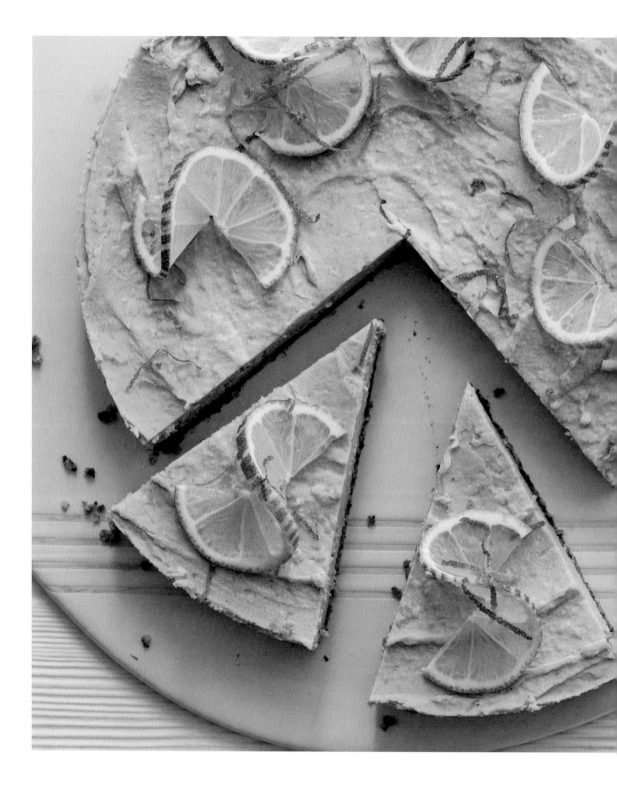

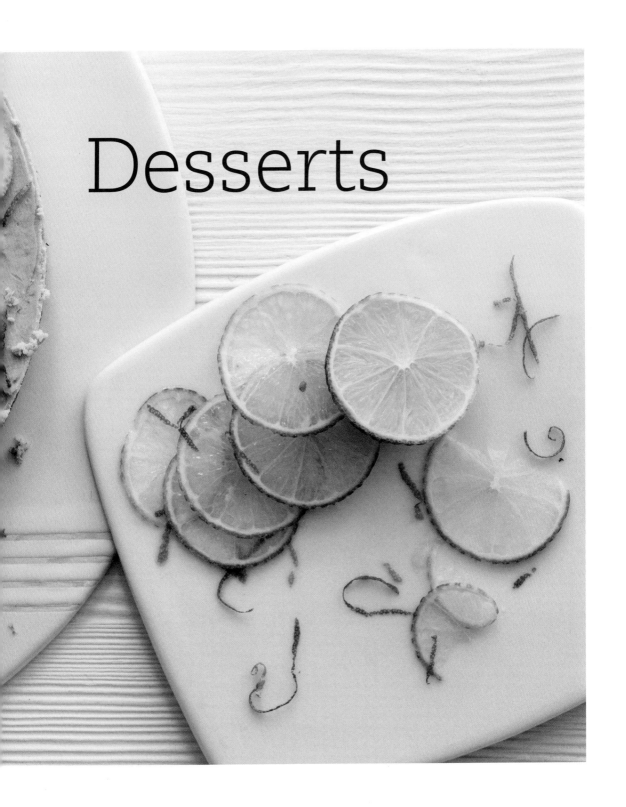

Desserts

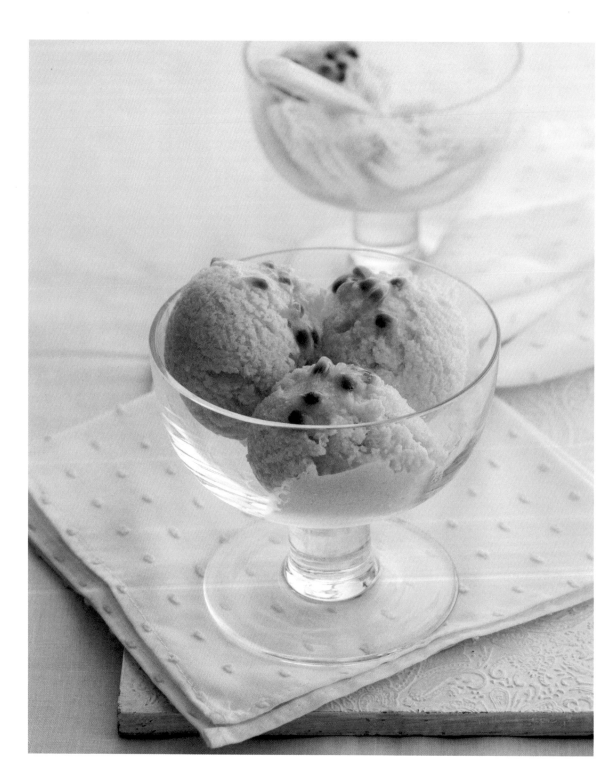

D E-F S-F

Passion Fruit Ice Cream

Rich, creamy and indulgent, this is a fabulous low-sugar ice cream. Use full-fat milk and Greek yogurt for a wonderfully rich texture. Studies have shown that you can boost your fertility by regularly including full-fat dairy products in your diet. The addition of yogurt also provides beneficial bacteria for supporting digestion and immune function.

5 passion fruit

200ml/7fl oz/scant 1 cup full-fat milk

300g/10½oz full-fat Greek yogurt

1 ripe mango, peeled, pitted and roughly chopped

½ tsp xanthan gum

1 tbsp honey

1 Scoop out the insides of the passion fruit. Strain the juice into a bowl and leave to one side. Reserve the seeds for decorating, if you like.

2 Put the milk, yogurt, mango, xanthan gum, honey and passion fruit juice in a blender or food processor and process until smooth.

3 Churn the mixture in an ice cream maker according to the manufacturer´s instructions. Alternatively, pour the mixture into a shallow container and freeze for 2–3 hours, stirring every hour to prevent ice crystals forming. Serve in scoops with a few seeds spooned over.

SERVES: 4 • PREPARATION TIME: 10 MINUTES, PLUS 2–3 HOURS FREEZING
NUTRITIONAL INFORMATION PER SERVING: PROTEIN 6.6G CARBOHYDRATE 15.8G, OF WHICH SUGARS 15.8G
FAT 9.8G, OF WHICH SATURATES 6.3G KCALS 178

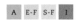

Acai Pomegranate Sorbet

A quick and easy sorbet that is packed with antioxidants and naturally sweet due to the cherries. The addition of coconut butter keeps the sorbet soft and creamy. Acai berries are a true superfood and one of the most nutritious foods of the Amazon, rich in protective anthocyanins, B-vitamins, minerals, fibre, protein and omega-3 fatty acids.

60g/2¼oz/1 cup unsweetened coconut flakes

¼ tsp xanthan gum

250ml/9fl oz/1 cup pomegranate juice

1 tbsp honey

1 tbsp coconut butter

a pinch of sea salt

1 tbsp acai berry powder

100g/3½oz/½ cup fresh or frozen pitted cherries

1 Put all the ingredients in a blender or food processor and process until smooth.

2 Pour the mixture into an ice cream maker and churn according to the manufacturer's instructions. Alternatively, pour the mixture into a shallow container and freeze for 4 hours, stirring every hour to prevent ice crystals forming.

3 To serve, remove the sorbet from the freezer about 15 minutes before required to allow it to soften slightly.

SERVES: 4 • PREPARATION TIME: 5 MINUTES, PLUS 4 HOURS FREEZING
NUTRITIONAL INFORMATION PER SERVING: PROTEIN 1.2G CARBOHYDRATE 15G, OF WHICH SUGARS 14.9G
FAT 10G, OF WHICH SATURATES 8G KCALS 155

E-F S-F S

Maca Lemon Iced Bars

This moreish, healthy bar is perfect for a sweet treat. The tangy lemon and maca cream combines beautifully with the chocolate nut base and it is delicious frozen or chilled. Maca is a root, grown in the Andes, which is incredibly nutrient-rich. Packed with vitamins and minerals, its health benefits have been long valued, and it is especially good at balancing the endocrine system.

225g/8oz/1¾ cups almonds

30g/1oz/2 tablespoons raw cacao powder

75g/2½oz/¾ cup raisins

juice and zest of 1 lemon

pomegranate seeds or berries, to serve

FILLING

100g/3½oz/⅔ cup cashew nuts

juice and zest of 3 lemons

5 tbsp honey

¼ tsp turmeric

1 tbsp maca powder

1 tbsp vanilla extract

a pinch of sea salt

3 tbsp coconut butter, melted

1 Line the base and sides of a 23 x 28cm/9 x 11in shallow traybake tin with cling film.

2 Put the almonds in a blender or food processor and process to form a flour-like mixture. Transfer to a mixing bowl, add the cacao powder and mix well.

3 Put the raisins and lemon juice and zest in the blender or food processor and process to form a thick paste. Add the paste to the bowl with the almonds and mix well to form a stiff dough.

4 Press the mixture into the base of the prepared traybake tin and press down firmly. Chill in the fridge while you make the filling.

5 Put the cashews, lemon juice, honey, turmeric, maca powder, vanilla and salt into the blender and process until creamy. Gradually pour in the melted coconut butter until it is all incorporated. Pour the filling over the base and freeze for 1–2 hours, or until firm.

6 Cut into 12 bars and keep in the fridge until ready to serve. Serve decorated with pomegranate seeds or berries.

Roasted Banana Caramel Mousse

Roasting bananas with their skins on creates a wonderful sweet caramelized flavour. The flesh is puréed with a healthy caramel-style sauce to create a thick mousse. Sweetened only with dates, this makes an irresistible healthy dessert. The pecans can be made in advance and stored in an airtight container. They make a delicious snack. One banana has an impressive 34 per cent of the recommended amount of vitamin B6, which is important for hormone balance, lowering homocysteine.

150g/5½oz/heaped ¾ cup soft pitted dates

2 bananas

2 tbsp almond butter

100ml/3½fl oz/generous ⅓ cup coconut milk

1 tsp vanilla extract

TOASTED NUTS

50g/1¾ oz/½ cup pecan nuts

1 tbsp maple syrup

1 tsp vanilla extract

½ tsp ground cinnamon

a pinch of sea salt

1 To make the toasted nuts, put the pecans in a bowl, cover with water and leave to soak for 2–4 hours, then drain.

2 Put the maple syrup, vanilla extract, cinnamon and salt in a bowl and mix well to combine. Add the drained pecans and toss them with the mixture to coat well.

3 Preheat the oven to 160°C/315°F/Gas 2–3 and line a baking tray with baking parchment. Spread the pecans on the prepared baking tray and bake for 20 minutes until crisp. Leave to cool, then roughly chop.

4 To make the mousse, put the dates in a bowl, cover with water and leave to soak for 20 minutes, then drain.

5 Meanwhile, preheat the oven to 200°C/400°F/Gas 6. Put the bananas on a baking sheet and bake for 20 minutes, until the skins are black. Leave to cool, then peel away the skins and place the flesh in a food processor or blender.

6 Add the drained dates to the food processor, along with the remaining ingredients and purée to form a thick mousse. Serve topped with the toasted pecans.

SERVES: 4 • PREPARATION TIME: 5 MINUTES, PLUS 2–4 HOURS SOAKING • COOKING TIME: 40 MINUTES
NUTRITIONAL INFORMATION PER SERVING: PROTEIN 4.4G CARBOHYDRATE 39.7G, OF WHICH SUGARS 38.2G
FAT 14G, OF WHICH SATURATES 1.3G KCALS 299

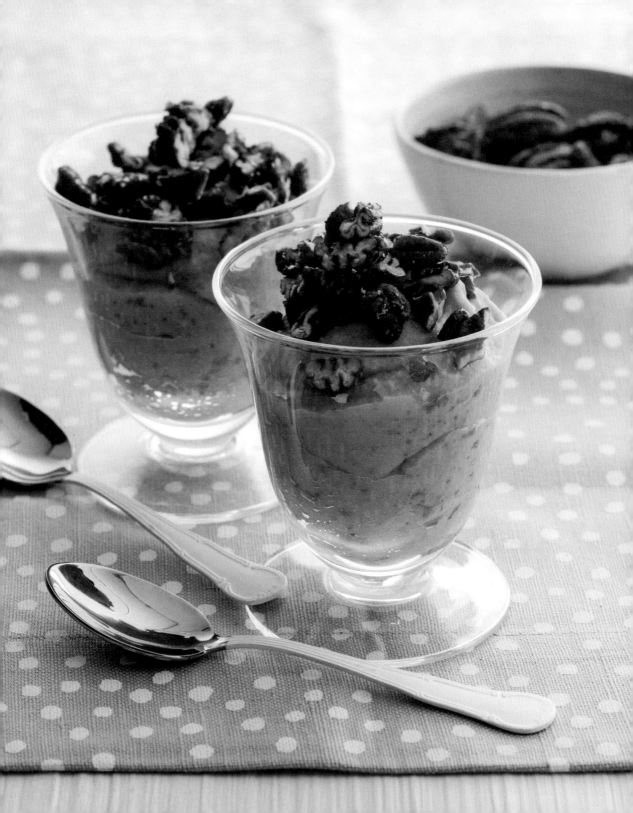

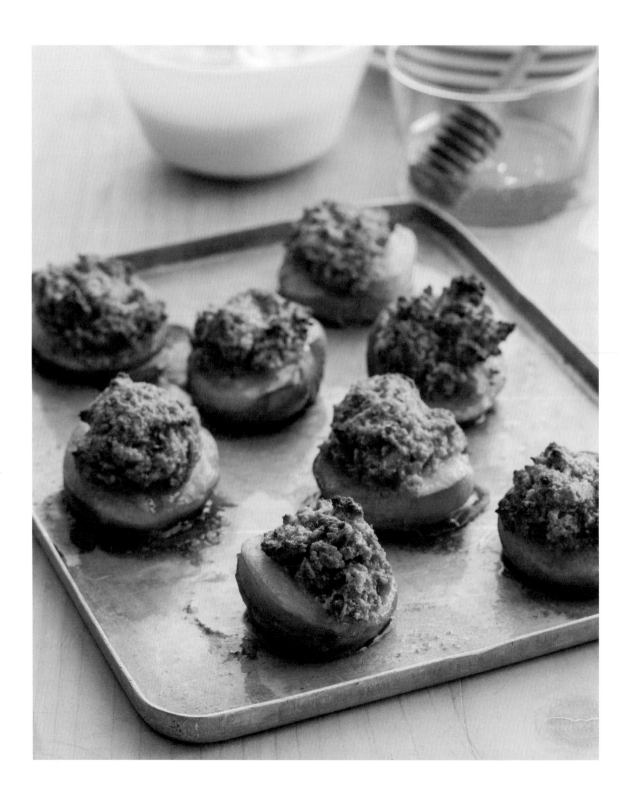

E-F S-F

Pistachio Honey Stuffed Peaches

A simple summery dessert – fresh peaches are topped with a delicious honey, pistachio crumb and baked until tender. Serve with a little yogurt or Mango Vanilla Cream (see page 62). You can also serve the peaches cold for breakfast or a snack option. Peaches are rich in vitamins C, E and A and chlorogenic acid, an antioxidant that helps neutralize harmful free radicals, protecting the body from damage and reducing inflammation.

115g/4oz/¾ cup shelled pistachio nuts

3 tbsp honey

4 firm, ripe peaches, halved and pitted

1 tablespoon butter

yogurt, to serve (optional)

1 Put the pistachios in a bowl, cover with water and leave to soak for at least 20 minutes, then drain, reserving the soaking water.

2 Put the drained pistachios in a food processor and add 2 tablespoons of the honey and a little of the reserved soaking water. Blend to form a thick paste, adding a little more water if needed.

3 Preheat the oven to 180°C/350°F/Gas 4. Put the halved peaches, cut side up, in a shallow roasting tin and dot with the butter. Spoon some of the pistachio paste into the centre of each peach half. Drizzle over the remaining honey and roast for 15 minutes, or until the peaches are just tender and lightly browned. Serve with a little yogurt, if you like.

SERVES: 4 • PREPARATION TIME: 5 MINUTES, PLUS AT LEAST 20 MINUTES SOAKING • COOKING TIME: 15 MINUTES
NUTRITIONAL INFORMATION PER SERVING: PROTEIN 5.9G CARBOHYDRATE 19.9G, OF WHICH SUGARS 19.7G
FAT 17G, OF WHICH SATURATES 2.8G KCALS 257

E-F S-F

Spiced Rice Pudding with Fruit Compôte

A delicious Indian-style rice pudding, which is rich and creamy. Using brown risotto or brown sushi rice means plenty of soluble fibre, vitamins and minerals, too. This is equally delicious served hot or cold for breakfast. Studies have shown that women eating a daily serving of full-fat dairy, such as milk, increase their chances of having a baby. Choose organic milk, which has a higher nutrient profile and also avoids unnecessary hormones, antibiotics and pesticides.

500ml/17fl oz/2 cups full-fat milk

2 cardamom pods, crushed

1 ball of preserved stem ginger, chopped

2 tbsp xylitol

zest of 1 orange

zest of 1 lemon

75g/2½oz/⅓ cup brown risotto rice, sushi rice or pudding rice

½ tsp rose water

FRUIT COMPOTE

8 ready-to-eat dried apricots, halved

3 tbsp apple juice

1 cinnamon stick, broken in half

2 tbsp chopped pistachio nuts

1 Preheat the oven to 150°C/300°F/Gas 2.

2 Heat the milk with the cardamom pods, ginger and xylitol in a saucepan over a medium heat. Remove from the heat and add the orange and lemon zest. Pour into a baking dish and stir in the rice. Cover with foil and bake for 1 hour 45 minutes, stirring occasionally. Remove from the oven and stir in the rose water. Return to the oven, uncovered, for a further 30 minutes, until lightly golden on top.

3 Meanwhile, make the fruit compôte. Put the apricots, apple juice and cinnamon stick in a saucepan over a medium heat and simmer gently for 5 minutes, then stir in the pistachios.

4 Serve the rice pudding topped with a spoonful of the compôte.

SERVES: 2 • PREPARATION TIME: 10 MINUTES • COOKING TIME: 2 HOURS 20 MINUTES
NUTRITIONAL INFORMATION PER SERVING: PROTEIN 13.9G CARBOHYDRATE 65.9G, OF WHICH SUGARS 37.3G
FAT 19.2G, OF WHICH SATURATES 7.3G KCALS 472

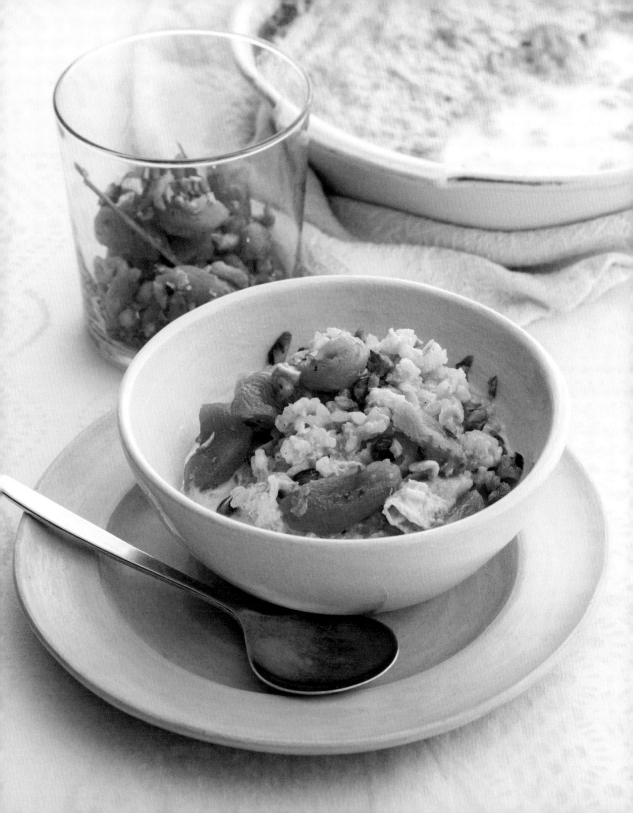

Lemon & Almond Cake

This dessert-style cake is simple to make and high in protein. It is wonderful served with yogurt and poached fruit. In addition to healthy fats and vitamin E, a quarter-cup of almonds contains almost a quarter of your daily magnesium requirements. Vitamin E is a powerful antioxidant and has been shown to help maintain healthy sperm.

2 lemons

2 clementines

olive oil, for greasing

250g/9oz/1⅔ cups almonds

4 eggs

1 tsp vanilla extract

100g/3½oz/½ cup xylitol or caster sugar

½ tsp sea salt

1 tsp baking powder

1 Wash the lemons and clementines and put them in a saucepan. Cover with water and bring to the boil over a medium heat. Turn the heat down, cover with a lid and leave to simmer gently for 1 hour, or until soft.

2 Preheat the oven to 180°C/350°F/Gas 4 and grease a 20cm/9in cake tin with olive oil. Put the almonds in a food processor and process to form a flour-like mixture.

3 Put the boiled citrus fruits in a food processor and blend until smooth. Add the eggs, vanilla extract, xylitol, almonds, salt and baking powder and process until well blended. Pour the batter into the prepared cake tin.

4 Bake for 45–50 minutes until a skewer inserted into the centre comes out clean. Leave to cool before removing from the tin.

SERVES: 10 • PREPARATION TIME: 10 MINUTES • COOKING TIME: 1 HOUR 50 MINUTES
NUTRITIONAL INFORMATION PER SERVING: PROTEIN 8G CARBOHYDRATE 12.6G, OF WHICH SUGARS 11.4G
FAT 16.2G, OF WHICH SATURATES 1.7G KCALS 213

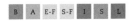

Key Lime Tart

The combination of sharp lime and rich creamy avocado makes an incredible creamy dessert. Coconut, cacao butter and lime are a winning combination and give this tart a light, tropical flavour. The tart can be frozen to create a wonderful iced dessert, too. Limes are an excellent source of vitamin C, which can enhance sperm quality, protecting sperm and the DNA within it from damage.

1 tbsp melted coconut oil, plus extra for greasing

115g/4oz/¾ cup almonds

30g/1oz/⅓ cup desiccated coconut

75g/2½oz/heaped ⅓ cup soft pitted dates, chopped

LIME FILLING

2 ripe avocados

6 tbsp maple syrup or honey

juice and zest of 2 limes, plus extra pared lime zest and lime slices, to decorate

1 tsp vanilla extract

75g/2½oz/5 tablespoons coconut butter, melted

75g/2½oz/5 tablespoons cacao butter, melted

1 Lightly grease a 20cm/8in springform cake tin with coconut oil. Put the almonds in a food processor and process to form a flour-like mixture. Add the remaining base ingredients and process until the mixture begins to stick together, adding a little water if needed. Press the mixture into the base of the prepared cake tin and chill in the fridge while you make the filling.

2 Put all the filling ingredients in a food processor or blender and process until smooth. Pour over the base and freeze for 2 hours until set, then transfer to the fridge until ready to serve. Decorate with lime zest and slices and serve.

Pictured on page 142

SERVES: 8 • PREPARATION TIME: 15 MINUTES, PLUS 2 HOURS FREEZING

NUTRITIONAL INFORMATION PER SERVING: PROTEIN 4.1G CARBOHYDRATE 14.7G, OF WHICH SUGARS 13.6G FAT 30.4G, OF WHICH SATURATES 15.4G KCALS 348

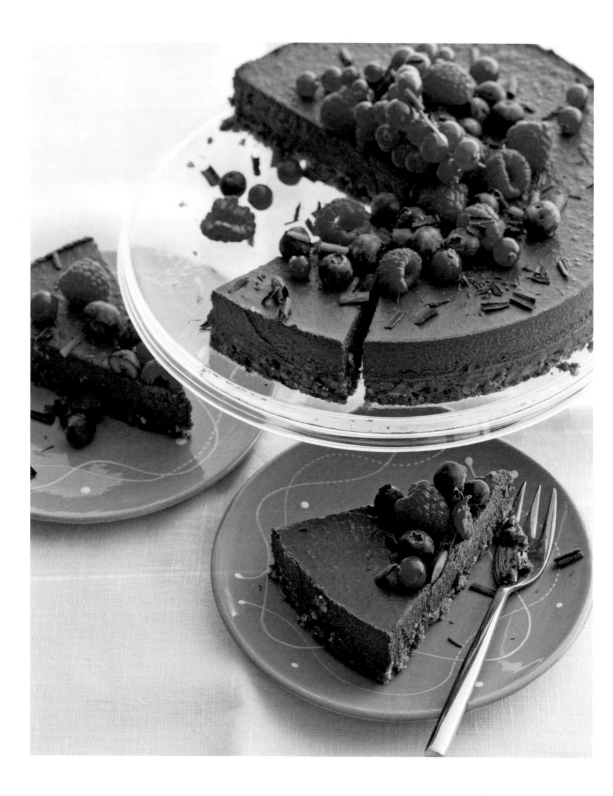

Chocolate Superfood Tart

Rich and indulgent, this amazing torte is perfect for a special occasion. It can be served frozen or chilled. Crammed with an array of superfoods and plenty of protein and healthy fats, it is a delicious way to energize the body. Raisins are a great source of instant energy and are packed with phenols – antioxidants that help prevent damage to cells in the body.

2 tbsp coconut oil, plus extra
   for greasing
125g/4½oz/1¼ cup pecan nuts
100g/3½oz/1 cup walnuts
2 tsp ground cinnamon
125g/4½oz/1 cup raisins
2 tsp maca powder

FILLING
250g/9oz/2⅔ cups cashew nuts
1 tbsp vanilla extract
1 tbsp lemon juice
100g/3½oz/heaped ¾ cup coconut
   butter, melted
1 tsp wheatgrass powder
1 tsp maca powder
160g/5¾oz/scant ½ cup honey or
   maple syrup
125ml/4fl oz/½ cup coconut water
   or water
60g/2¼oz/½ cup raw cacao powder
fresh berries and chocolate
   shavings, to serve

1 Grease a 20cm/8in springform cake tin with coconut oil. Put all the ingredients for the base in a food processor and pulse until well combined. Press the mixture into the base of the prepared cake tin and and chill in the fridge while you make the filling.

2 Put all the filling ingredients in a food processor or blender and process until smooth. Pour over the base and freeze for 2 hours until set, then transfer to the fridge until ready to serve. Decorate with fresh berries and chocolate shavings and serve.

SERVES: 10 • PREPARATION TIME: 15 MINUTES, PLUS 2 HOURS FREEZING
NUTRITIONAL INFORMATION PER SERVING: PROTEIN 8.8G CARBOHYDRATE 29.1G, OF WHICH SUGARS 21.8G
FAT 40G, OF WHICH SATURATES 14.3G KCALS 513

Index

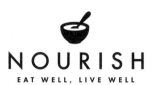

NOURISH
EAT WELL, LIVE WELL

We hope you've enjoyed this Nourish book. Here at Nourish we're all about wellbeing through food and drink – irresistible dishes with a serious good-for-you factor. If you want to eat and drink delicious things that set you up for the day, suit any special diets, keep you healthy and make the most of what you can afford, we've got some great ideas to share with you. Come over to our blog for wholesome recipes and fresh inspiration – nourishbooks.com